Laboring Well
A labor nurse shares insights from 10,000 births

by

Elizabeth Allen RN MN

TELEMACHUS PRESS

Dearest Brittany,
Many blessings on the pursuit
of your most cherished dreams!
Praying you have the chance to
care for laboring women one
day. You will be
such a blessing
to them!
In Him,
Elizabeth

LABORING WELL

Cover Designed by Telemachus Press, LLC

Cover Art:
Copyright © 126859809/Zoonar/Thinkstock

Interior images by
  Elizabeth Allen
  Ryan McCarthy

Permission for images on file

Visit the author website
http://www.laboringwell.com

Published by Telemachus Press, LLC
http://www.telemachuspress.com

ISBN: 978-1-938701-72-6 (eBook)
ISBN: 978-1-938701-73-3 (Paperback)

Version 2012.11.21

Printed in the United States of America

10 9 8 7 6 5 4 3 2 1

Contents

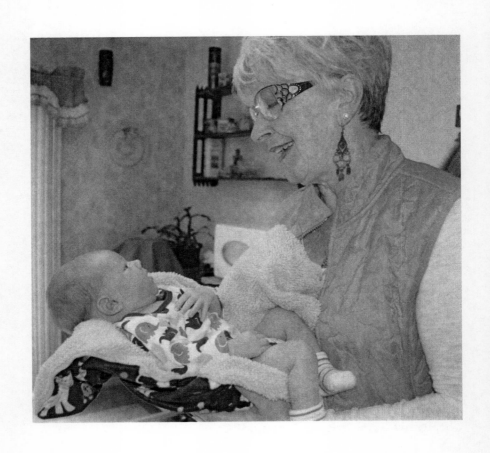

For mom
with love

Laboring Well
A labor nurse shares insights from 10,000 births

Introduction

Preparing to have your baby is a very exciting time. You have so many thoughts and feeling swirling through your head and trying to sort through them all can be overwhelming. Being the information age there are a lot of ideas and opinions out there (including those of your mother, your mother-in-law, your best friend, and 500 women on the internet!)

How do you know what to hang onto and what to let go of? What to believe and what to question? Ultimately we all want to make good decisions and bring forth a happy healthy baby. If you want an insider's perspective on labor then this book is for you.

Labor is simple really. It's the process by which your body works to get the baby out—and for some of you, this is all you care to know. And that's just fine. Truthfully, I don't believe that you need to read this book—or any book—in order to have a good birth. Your doctor or midwife and nurse will know exactly how to take care of you and help you through your journey. But, if you have questions or are someone who likes to explore every angle, then hopefully this book will offer you food for thought.

Every labor is unique, so my first word of encouragement is *don't compare yourself!* Women compare themselves all the time whether we're honest about it or not (from clothes and shoes, to husbands and kids …). But when it comes to labor, comparing yourself to others is a big no-no. You are unique, your baby is unique and your labor will be uniquely yours. Many women set themselves up for unnecessary grief by silently comparing themselves. Please don't be one of them.

In order to talk about labor, we'll have to cover all possibilities. It's true that some women have the baby come out and *don't* experience labor. That's called an elective cesarean section. Then there are those who *labor* and also experience surgical birth. That's called an *unexpected* cesarean section. There are also women who *schedule* a cesarean section and end up experiencing some degree of labor (these women find this a real bummer!)

And of course there are many women who still have good old fashioned vaginal births.

Vaginal birth also comes in a wide array of styles. Some labors are long, some are short; some babies need help coming into the world, and some catapult out before we can even put our gloves on. There are so many possible scenarios—and I'm guessing that you have your favorite! This is because, even though labor is a simple concept, in truth, it's a wonderful, amazing, and unpredictable phenomenon. We'll explore each scenario and try to understand a bit more about why each one happens.

I hope that you're a first-time mom because I'm writing this book especially for you. First-time moms are special and unique—in more ways than one. You're unique physically because your body hasn't gone through the process of birth before. And you tend to be unique emotionally and psychologically because your *mind* hasn't gone through the process of birth before. For both reasons, I love caring for first-time moms. I love the unique challenge—both physically and psychologically—that the first-time mom package presents.

But, maybe you're a second or third time mom who's now wondering what insights about labor you wish you would have known the first time around. This book is for you too. Of course, if you're having your eighth baby, you could be writing this book! But whatever your story, I'm so happy to have you joining me in this journey.

It's also possible that you're taking a peek into this book because you're just plain curious to know who in the world I am and what qualifies me to write a book about labor. Well, I'm glad you asked. In all honesty, even after 20 years of caring for women in labor I'm still learning. Labor, as simple as it sounds on paper, is a really big topic. When you start experiencing birth you soon begin to realize that there's more to learn than meets the eye. There are so many possible scenarios that it could take a lifetime to learn about them all. But, in my 20 years I've seen my fair share: the good, the bad, the ugly … the normal, the paranormal and then some!

In those 20 years, I've had the indescribable privilege of being a Labor and Delivery nurse and experiencing birth on three very unique continents. Ten thousand births is a conservative estimate. Between seeing, doing and talking about deliveries, the actual number is probably closer to 20 or 30 thousand. And even so, I still haven't seen it all.

My first birth experience was in Kenya where I worked one summer at a small rural hospital. This was the "no frills but lots of thrills" approach to childbirth. We had babies arriving before the midwife could get to the bedside and one who couldn't even wait to get to the bed and delivered in the grass just outside the main gate. (Now for some of you this is your idea of the perfect birth, but I don't recommend it. Not when our precious infant took a nose dive into the rich African soil and ingested a mouthful of dirt!).

What a profound difference all of that was from my next birth experience at a large teaching and research hospital. Here we had all the gizmos and gadgets. Childbirth in this environment was a scientific endeavor with rationale and research to back up every decision and movement we made. I learned a lot during my tenure there; the most important being that *there's a lot to learn.*

After working there for three years experiencing some of the most interesting and challenging obstetrical cases known to man, I was ready for a change. So I packed my bags and moved to the heart of the Islamic world to deliver babies for the Bedouin. (By "change" my family thought I meant orthopedics.)

I spent nearly two years in the Middle East working in a very busy Labor and Delivery unit. For those of you familiar with terms like *census* and *space capacity* you'll appreciate the thrill of our daily work life. In six small labor rooms we delivered an average of 20 babies every day! (In the hospital where I currently work we deliver 12 babies on average every day in 10 labor rooms—and this is considered busy.) The advantage that we had in the Middle East was that our Bedouin women were quite experienced at giving birth and so were very efficient. Typically, a Bedouin woman gives birth to 10, 12 or even 15 babies before all is said and done, so people came and went very quickly.

This a simple book really, for I'm a simple, straightforward sort of person. This is the "nuts and bolts," no frills version of *how to have a good birth*. An honest, from my heart, conversation with you about what you need to know—and *don't* need to know—as you approach your labor.

If I could, I'd prefer to sit with you over a cup of coffee and chat with you about your thoughts and feelings, fears and ideas. Then I'd know more about who you are and where you're coming from. But, alas, this is a limitation. Writing—and reading—a book is a one way conversation. But

I do want to try to get you involved and, in places, have tried to help you engage with me about some really important points.

I say this a bit tongue-in-cheek, because if you knew me you would know that every "point" is important to me. Like many labor nurses, I'm a bit opinionated and profoundly passionate about the topic of labor. And as I've browsed the market for books on this subject, it seems to me that there's a regrettable shortage of books written by labor nurses. We who are laboring in the trenches with laboring women have so much to share.

Why don't nurses write books? Well, my best guess is that, like everyone, we're very busy people. It's the age-old excuse though for not taking advantage of opportunities or pursing dreams. But nurses should write books! We have *great* stories to tell, but herein lies the dilemma. In the "telling" we run the risk of betraying the privacy of our beloved patients. And privacy laws in healthcare are sacred. Thus we keep our stories locked inside the rich warehouse of our memories, never to be told or enjoyed by others. This is a shame. Many of our stories carry with them rich nuggets of wisdom that could be of great benefit to the lives of others. And also, they're just really great stories!

I share a few of my stories with you here for the purpose of bringing my "points" to life. But please know that each story has been effectively altered so as to guard the privacy of my patients and their families. And all names are fictitious. Any presumed association is purely coincidental. Birth stories share many similarities; if they didn't, women would find no enjoyment in sharing them with each other!

Another reason that nurses should write books is because we're the ones doing a large portion of the work. I know that sounds like a no-brainer, but you would be surprised by how many people *think* they know the work of the trenches, but have never actually worked in the trenches. I'm sure it's like any industry. Everyone outside your job thinks they know all about it—how to do it, how much time you need to do it, the best way to do it, and so on. But they don't actually do it. Nurses have a unique perspective and a unique experience—because we're there. It's our "lived reality" to use a favorite modern phrase.

Nurses are powerful people. We make a lot of decisions within a prescribed set of guidelines. I once polled a large group of family and friends and discovered that they believed that nurses only and always followed doctor's orders. And to a certain extent this is true. But what was missing in their understanding was that there are many decisions that nurses make that are not specifically stated in an order.

For example, Labor and Delivery nurses decide when or when not to remove the monitoring belts, the blood pressure cuff, or the oxytocin. We decide when to check for cervical dilation or encourage a soak in the tub. Labor nurses interpret how the baby is coping with labor and determine the best strategy to employ if baby needs some help.

Labor nurses decide when to call the doctor or midwife with concerns or issues. We decide how things are progressing and what strategy to try to promote the process. Labor nurses also decide when it's time for medication or an epidural. And we're the ones who decide when it's time to call the doctor or midwife for delivery—not too late, and not too soon. Our training and experience guides these decisions.

We coach, counsel and comfort. We guide the plan of care based upon the unique set of variables that are presented to us. We don't treat you all the same, because you are all different and have different needs and ideas. We give input related to positioning strategies and how things are working for you. We do a lot of teaching about labor, breathing and relaxation. And most importantly, we assure your loved ones that "this is all normal."

There are a lot of people out there who have strong opinions on the subject of labor. You may be one of them. Access to the internet gives us the opportunity to tap into conversations from every corner of the globe. Some conversations are worth tapping into, and some should raise our concerns. How do you know who to believe and who to question? Well, ultimately we choose to believe the people that we trust. The truth is though that some people are more worthy of your trust than others. The criteria you choose for placing your trust in someone will be uniquely yours. But, it's my hope that after reading this book you'll have more tools for making choices based upon sound, current, and common sense evidence.

So let's begin this journey. And just so that we're all speaking the same language, let's start by exploring some basic definitions: like *what is labor really?*

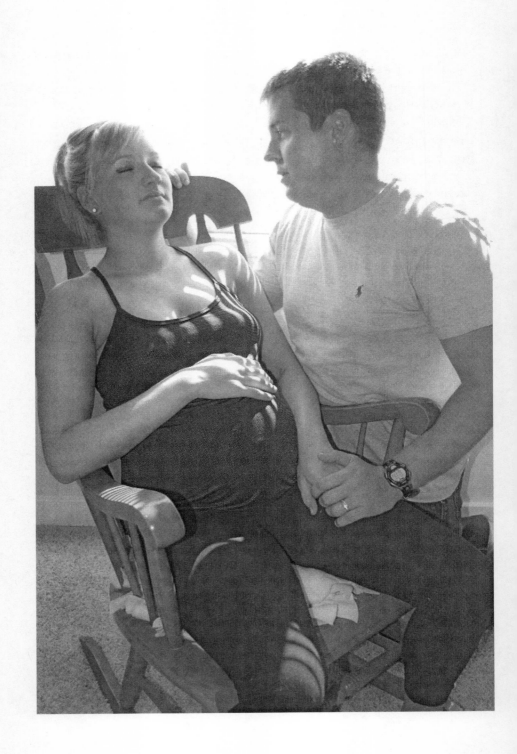

Prelude
A day at the office

I could hear the pounding as I walked down the hall. It sounded a bit like some ancient drumming ritual. And with the pounding came a chorus of shouting "ONE, TWO, THREE …"

I gathered my thoughts and quietly entered the room. I surveyed the scene before me, unnoticed by the flushed group of people scattered in various positions and states of undress about the room. The mother-to-be was sitting straddled over a large ball pounding the bed with her fist; her husband and companions shouting and pounding in unison with her.

I watched quietly for a few moments, processing the information I just got from the previous nurse.

As a labor nurse I see a lot of things and have come to recognize that sometimes my role is a bit precarious. People don't know me when I walk through the door and in some cases aren't overly interested. That's ok. I'm not there to earn a popularity award; I'm there to perform a privileged job. Sometimes though I have a bit of work to do as the new person coming into an established situation. Women in labor have asked a lot of questions and have people they trust to give them answers, and one of those people isn't automatically me.

The atmosphere in the room of the pounder was a little unique. Women typically like things quiet and peaceful during labor, maybe with soft music playing in the background. A relaxed, calm environment often helps promote a relaxed, calm mommy. Women can do whatever they like when they're in labor as far as I'm concerned. The questions filtering through my mind weren't related to her unique choice of labor strategies, but to whether her strategy was *working* for her.

"What do you mean was her strategy *working for her*?" you ask. Some of you may be wondering if it was right to critique. Isn't anything a mom chooses to do or believe ok? Well, not always. Not if you want to have a vaginal birth that is. Labor either happens, or it doesn't. Now the *journey* of each labor will be unique, but the *mechanisms* of each labor will be the same. Sometimes certain behaviors and strategies actually work against the process. One of the biggest differences between women in regards to labor is how quickly it all happens—*if* it happens.

As a labor nurse, *working* to me means that my client is getting somewhere; that her labor is going forward. I think that we would all agree that ultimately *getting somewhere* is the desirable thing. No one would want this poor woman stuck at 7cm forever. And this was the situation with my new client. I knew from report that she hadn't made any progress past 7cm in nearly 3 hours. Thus, another issue before me (on top of being the newcomer who no one trusts yet) is the fact that I have a client who's fading fast—emotionally and physically—and stuck at 7cm.

My new mom was brave and strong. Her fortitude and spunk were admirable. This was her first baby and she was a week overdue. Her water broke early Tuesday morning and mild irregular contractions soon followed. She got to the hospital at 7am, and because she had no issues was allowed to go home and let labor kick in on its own. Eventually, twelve hours after her water broke, labor did indeed "kick in" and she returned to the hospital at 8pm.

Twenty-six hours after her water broke (Wednesday morning), I walked through the door of her room. She'd been working hard in spite of little sleep and slow progress. Her first cervical exam was at 11pm the evening before when she was found to be 4cm dilated, 90% effaced, and minus 1 station. At 5am she was 7cm, and at 8am her cervix was still a disheartening 7cm. For a woman desiring natural childbirth, this news is hard to take.

Labor nurses must balance many things: hopes and dreams, the well-being of two clients (one seen and one unseen), and reality. I began to suspect that maybe the whole pounding phenomenon might be contributing to the situation, but I sat and watched for a while. I didn't want to barge in and completely upset the apple cart, not initially anyway. I calmly asked some questions, *between* contractions. The hoopla that each contraction provoked prevented anyone from hearing anything beyond the pounding!

It was easy to see, as I watched her work her way through contractions, that she was tense and anxious. Her back was as ridged as a flag pole and her shoulders nearly touched her ears. Between contractions she fought back tears. If I was going to interject new ideas into this situation I'd have to do so very gently.

There wasn't anything overly unusual about what was happening, so no reason to panic. But because I felt concerned about her ability to make it to her goal of a non-medicated, natural birth, I knew that we needed to do something different or she was going to run out of energy before she ran out of labor. We needed to find out soon if she was really stuck at 7cm or just experiencing technical difficulties. If her next exam didn't show some change, her doctor would likely recommend trying some oxytocin to help strengthen the contractions, or an epidural to help relax the pelvis.

When I coach someone in labor I've learned never to ask "do you want to try …?" because the answer is typically "no." Instead it seems to work better if I take a positive, more assertive approach like: "Mary, let's try _____." This conveys the message that I have confidence in the new trick even if I have no idea how it will work for her! The idea is that sometimes doing *anything* different can help push labor forward. Quite often women in an intense phase of labor find one position that they like best and cling to it for dear life. Such was the case with my pounder.

Thankfully my new patient was the open minded sort. As a group we coaxed Mary to try the swaying technique. (As much as I wanted to coax her into the tub, she'd already spent enough time in water to have permanently shriveled feet). We raised the bed to about waist height, and instead of sitting on the ball I had Mary lean across it as it rested on the bed. Most importantly, we experimented with a new breathing technique (thus gloriously abandoning the pounding and shouting regimen!)

I leaned over the bed next to Mary and asked her to breathe with me. I demonstrated for her how to blow out and relax her shoulders simultaneously. I didn't care if she took a breath in through her nose or in through her mouth; I just wanted to see those shoulders come down. As she blew the air hard out of her mouth I gently touched her shoulders, asking her to bring them down. I stood close by and breathed with her through each contraction, reminding her to loosen her shoulders with each breath. It didn't take long for her to get the hang of it and things began to change.

Next we spent time helping Mary soak up the wonderful rest periods *between* contractions. This was how she would regain some of her mental and physical energy. Granted the "rest periods" weren't very long, but they were critical for both Mary and her baby.

We encouraged her to sway from side to side with each contraction and to let her hips go loose. I rubbed her low back and in time felt much of the tension subside. One contraction at a time she rocked and swayed. In time the tense look disappeared and a quiet determination filled her face.

The whole room gained a peaceful sort of quiet. No one talked, no one moved. We waited. And watched. We were seeing a marvelous transformation happen before our eyes. And then it came again. Another powerful surge of energy from the center of her abdomen. It gripped her entire belly with powerful force. She groaned and moved of her own volition. This time she bent her knees and sagged down the side of the bed. When the contraction ended she rested over the ball and quietly swayed some more. Even with her eyes closed Mary had a steady, resigned look about her. As I watched I felt really optimistic that we would find some change in her cervix with the next exam.

About 40 minutes later, I saw another subtle change come over Mary. With each contraction she seemed to stop breathing altogether. The groaning stopped and even though I knew she was contracting, she was quiet as a lamb. She seemed to be gently, quietly pushing down—like she wasn't sure she should, but as if something was propelling her in that direction.

Since I hadn't examined her cervix yet, I asked if I could. Women often feel an urge to push when there's still a lot of cervix left. In some cases, especially for first-time moms, bearing down on the cervix can be problematic: like catching your thumb between the tabletop and a hammer. No one wants a swollen cervix.

On exam, Mary was now 9cm dilated and the baby's head was at +2 station. This news brought shouts of joy from around the room and renewed hope and determination on the face of my brave patient. We were so close now to entering the pushing stage, and with that a whole new world of sensation. Feeling an intense amount of pressure and a growing urge to push, I encouraged her to do some light, patterned breathing until the remaining rim of cervix retracted. Now also seemed like a good time to encourage a trip to the bathroom because sitting on the toilet does wonders for coaxing that last bit of cervix away!

Thirty minutes later Mary was fully dilated and began pushing in earnest. Ninety minutes later she brought forth her first-born son and wrapped him tightly in her grateful arms.

It's all about a happy ending.

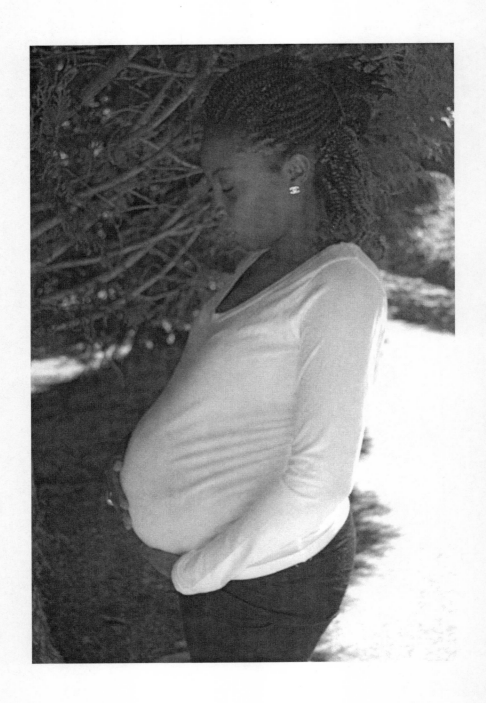

Chapter One
Understanding labor

The anatomy of labor

Women come in many different packages—physically and emotionally (like this surprises any of you!) Physically you're fairly similar, but psychologically, you're as different as oranges and apples. Good labor nurses get into the minds of their clients. I've always said if you like psychology, go into Labor and Delivery. Labor is an intensely psychological, emotional, dramatic journey, and good labor nurses, midwives and physicians understand this.

As we talk about labor in all its glory, I'll also give you a peek into the mind of your ***provider*** and help you understand the answers to questions like:

- What did she mean when she said that my cervix was favorable?
- What did he mean when she said that I'm not in labor yet?
- Why did she send me home when I'm having so many painful contractions?
- What does it mean to be "stuck"?

So to get us started thinking on the same page and speaking the same language, let's begin with a good working definition. And let's start at the beginning:

What is labor?

LABOR IS:
Progressive cervical change in the presence of regular painful contractions

Well, outside of the fact that this sounds like something fresh out of a textbook, it gets right to the point. But what does it mean? Let's put it another way: labor is not a *number*—like 3 or 4—it's a **rate of change**. For some reason this concept can be a bit confusing—even for those of us who work in the business! I think this is because we still want to define labor as "pain," "contractions," "days," or even "tears." Moms tend to define labor in those terms because that's all they have to go by, but those things don't necessarily mean that you're in labor.

Labor is *progressive cervical change*. Progressive does ***not*** mean that last week you saw you're doctor or midwife and you were one centimeter dilated, and this week you're two. Progressive means *hourly*. When you're in good labor, your cervix will dilate about one centimeter an hour—give or take an hour.

Hold tightly to this definition because I'm going to quiz you down the road to see how well you have it locked down. But before we start working with our definition of labor, it would be good for us to have a brief conversation about *anatomy*. You may not even be sure what a "cervix" is and I don't want to make any assumptions! So here we go. If you're squeamish, I hope you're sitting in your favorite chair.

Your uterus (or womb) is the place where your baby lives and grows. When you're *not* pregnant, your uterus is a small pear shaped organ located in the lower part of your abdomen just behind your bladder. The uterus is an *amazing* organ. It has the ability to stretch many times its original size, and then go back again shortly after delivery. Think of the stories you've heard of women who've been pregnant with 2, 3 or even 8 babies! The uterus can stretch to accommodate all of these babies.

Dangling off the lower part of the uterus is the cervix. You could say that the cervix is the door to the womb, locking the baby in during pregnancy and opening to let the baby out during labor. It's really a part of the uterus but functions a lot differently. If you pucker up your lips and push them out for a kiss, you have a rough picture of what your cervix looks like. It has a tiny opening in the center that has the capacity to open really wide. (If you're still puckering up for that kiss, open your lips really wide now!). If you could look at it for yourself you would see that it looks like a very tiny pink donut.

The cervix is also an amazing organ. Actually, I originally wanted to title this book *"It's All About the Cervix"*—because, well, it is! Labor, in terms of definitions, is all about the cervix. But here I am, straying off into the definition of labor again. Once we finish anatomy lesson we'll talk more about what the amazing cervix does during labor (it's very exciting!)

This might come as a surprise to some of you, but did you know that you have *three* openings down there? You have your **vagina**, which is the pathway to the cervix and uterus, your **urethra**, which is where the urine comes out, and your **rectum**, where the stool comes out.

The vagina is the middle opening. It's a fairly long, tube-like pathway and is surrounded by layers of muscle. Of course everyone is different—not in terms of anatomy per se, but in terms of the particulars. Some vaginas are longer, some are shorter, some muscles are tighter, some are more flexible (notice I didn't use the word *flabby*—though if you want an easy delivery, there's nothing wrong with flabby!)

When the baby comes out of the uterus he or she has a journey to make: through the cervix, down the vagina, and over the **perineum** (aka your bottom). This is the last body part that we're going to talk about. The perineum is the area between the lower part of your vagina and your rectum. The muscles from the vagina are also part of the perineum. This area stretches when the baby's head comes into the vagina and pushes on it from the inside. This area has a lot of stretching to do in order to get the vagina open enough to let the baby's head out. The baby won't come out until the perineum stretches enough to let it—and this can take a while.

Can you see now that if the tissues are more pliable it will take less work to get them to stretch? (This might be an "ah-ha" moment for some of you who've been told that strong bottom muscles help you have a better birth!)

Ripe as a peach

Have you ever picked fruit? Apples? Strawberries?? Which is easier to pick—green fruit or ripe fruit? Even if you've never picked fruit, I think you can probably guess that ripe fruit is easier to pick than green fruit. Ripe fruit is soft and *ready* while green fruit is hard and stubborn. When a strong wind comes along it knocks ripe fruit right off the branch; but try picking green fruit and you get the whole branch!

Your cervix is like fruit. Before you go into labor it goes through a **ripening** process. It *must* go through a ripening process or you'll never get that baby out! Like fruit, the process of cervical ripening takes time. Ripening can start as early as 36 or 37 weeks, but more commonly at about 38, maybe 39 weeks of pregnancy. Some women experience ripening *very* early in their pregnancy. This is a complication of pregnancy called premature labor and we don't want this for you (more on this in Chapter Eleven). Others won't get any ripening until closer to or after their due date. And some women never get any ripening. There are so many possible scenarios.

But let's pretend that everything is normal and your pregnancy has been textbook. As you approach your due date your cervix gets *ready*. Every cervix gets ready by *ripening* and every cervix ripens at a different pace.

What's involved in ripening since it's so central to the process of labor?

When the cervix ripens it begins to get soft. Normally the cervix is about 2 inches long, feels firm, and the donut hole in the center is closed. (Of course it's not *completely* closed because if that were the case you'd never get pregnant!) But from our perspective, it remains closed, or tightly shut, during your pregnancy to lock the baby into the uterus. As your due date approaches it begins to loosen up and soften in preparation for labor.

Once your cervix is soft it then begins to *thin*. This means that it loses its length: slowly shrinking over time from 2 inches to 1 inch to ½ an inch and so on, until it's *paper-thin*. This process of thinning is called *effacement*. Most of the effacing process happens during ripening phase *before* real labor starts. The last little bit, getting it to the paper thin stage, typically happens during labor. Typically, by the time most women are 5 or 6 centimeters, the cervix has thinned 100% of the way.

The other thing that the cervix does about 2 to 7 days before you go into labor is rotate forward. When you're not in labor your cervix points toward your bum, but as you approach your labor is moves forward to point straight down your vagina. The baby's head plays a role in the process of getting the cervix ready and in position. As the baby descends it pushes the cervix before it. When we examine you we feel all of these things. We use all of this information to help us guess how close you are to having your baby.

Quite often ripening happens without you even knowing it. Many people (moms as well as care takers) mistake ripening phase for labor phase. This is because you might have some mild irregular contractions during ripening phase to help the process along. Some women are aware of contractions, some are not. They can be so mild that you hardly notice them.

It's important to remember the fruit analogy at this point. If you think about how long it takes fruit to ripen you can appreciate how long it may take for your cervix to ripen. (As I sit here on this lovely September afternoon in the wilds of the Pacific Northwest I have a real appreciation for this. My beautiful tomatoes have been lime green for 3 weeks now and I'm beginning to wonder if they'll ripen before Christmas!) You may feel the same way about your cervix one of these days too!

If you're a first-time mom your cervix will typically ripen slowly over the 2 weeks before your due date. This means that if your provider examines your cervix you will hear him or her say nice things like "oh, it's getting soft," or "your cervix is quite favorable." They may even give you more objective data like "your cervix is 50% effaced now," or "you're dilated to 1 centimeter." None of these changes though mean that you're in labor. They simply mean that your cervix is doing the very necessary job of *ripening*. And the more ripening you get before you go into labor the better. Often the degree of ripening you get before true labor starts relates to the length of your labor. So pray for ripening!

Women who've had babies before have a real advantage in the cervix department. Their cervixes tend to be softer naturally because they've been through the process before. This is why women who've had babies usually have shorter labors. Because it's all about the cervix! And a ripe cervix is an efficient cervix. (I've known second and third time moms who ripened to 4 or even 5 centimeters *before* they were even in labor. If 80% of the work is done before labor even starts, you can see how that may contribute to a shorter labor.)

Let's talk about how contractions fit into the picture now. It makes sense that if the cervix is soft and thin it will respond better to the power of contractions. In what way do we want the cervix to respond to contractions? By opening so that the baby can come out. The door must open, and the baby must come out—if you want a vaginal birth that is!

When the cervix opens we say it's *dilating*. We measure dilation in centimeters. Like effacement, measuring changes in the cervix is done by putting one or two fingers into the cervix and feeling it. It's not very scientific, so don't be surprised if two different examiners say two different things. Don't worry about this though. Since we're more concerned about determining **change**, the actual number or percentage is less important.

The cervix dilates from zero to 10 centimeters. That's how we describe it. But I think if we describe it in terms of a percentage it makes more sense. In order to get the baby out the cervix needs to be 100% open. Ten centimeters is 100% open. That means that when we reach in and examine the situation, we can't feel the cervix anymore. It's completely gone. Well it doesn't actually disappear. More correctly, it retracts upward as the baby comes downward.

The reason I like the percentage description better is because I've been asked by couples why the baby can't be born vaginally if the cervix is only open to 9 centimeters—especially if the baby is small. The answer is that the cervix is an obstruction to the baby and the baby cannot come out unless the cervix is out of the way—or 100% gone.

The power of contractions and the pressure of the baby's head make the cervix open. Think about picking fruit again. The power of your hand on the fruit is like the power of the contraction on the cervix. Like the fruit, the cervix responds favorably to the power placed upon it—if it's ripe. When the cervix is ripe it dilates, when it isn't ripe, it doesn't. (You'll never think of apples the same way again!)

Here's a real life example demonstrating what I mean. Many of you have probably heard of the hormone oxytocin. It's a substance that makes the uterus contract. I can make someone contract all day by giving them oxytocin through an I.V. line and never see any change in the cervix. I can even make someone contract every 2 minutes for 12 hours and see no change in the cervix.

How can this be? *Because this cervix wasn't ripe and thus wouldn't respond.* The good news is that if the cervix isn't responding, mom typically isn't feeling much discomfort. Of course this is also bad news if our goal is to promote labor! The pain of labor comes from the fact that the cervix is responding to the power of contractions and making progressive change. Thus the old saying is true: no pain, no gain. But the friendly corollary is also true: the more pain, the more gain. This is how it is in our world of birth.

So to summarize, ripening is everything if you want labor to happen. Ripening is how your cervix prepares for labor by getting soft and thin and it takes a long time. Ripening can also be *dilating*—but very slow dilating. Consider Sally's situation:

- At 38 weeks her cervix was 1 centimeter dilated and 50% effaced
- At 39 weeks her cervix is now 2 centimeters dilated and 80% effaced

These changes don't reflect labor, they reflect *ripening* because they're happening very slowly and don't fit the definition of *progressive*. Sally is getting good ripening and her cervix is *favorable* for labor, but she's not in labor yet. The most favorable factor of her exam is the *thinning* part. Most women *thin* before they *dilate*. A cervix that's thin is a cervix that can respond to contractions. We all get excited about dilation, but you should be ecstatic if you're getting good thinning.

Our friend Sally could stay at 2 centimeters for another week or two, or she may get even more thinning or more dilating before real labor starts. Anything is possible. ***But she isn't in labor until contractions are coming about every 2 to 3 minutes and her cervix is progressively changing.***

Women are hormonal
And thank God! Without hormones we don't function. Without insulin our cells would die of starvation. Without adrenaline we wouldn't be able to respond to trouble. And without progesterone we can't secure the baby in the uterus.

Labor is also hormonally driven. Actually, we don't quite know exactly what gets the process going, but we have a few ideas, and most of them are related to hormones[1].

The main point of this discussion is to tell you that there's little you can do to get labor going if the hormones haven't decided to kick in yet. There are a variety of ideas and myths out there, but the best strategy is *patience*. We'll talk more about ideas for getting labor going in Chapter Eight.

Patience is a virtue

If you're like me, patience doesn't come naturally. I don't want things now, I want them yesterday! But when it comes to labor, patience is everything. (It's how God prepares you for parenthood!)

Getting into labor can take time. There's this weird, frustrating grey zone before real labor starts that can be very tiring and confusing. Many people call it *false labor* but I really don't like that term because it's sounds so defeating. Here you are contracting your heart out, getting excited about the birth of your baby and your nurse tells you "I'm sorry Mrs. Jones; you're only in false labor. Come back when the contractions are closer." It's very discouraging!

It's true; we who work in this business seem a little hard hearted sometimes. But there's no point in being dishonest with you and admitting you to Labor and Delivery if you're not in labor. And being admitted when you're not in labor may present some disadvantages.

So what do we really mean by "false labor"? Technically this just means that when we examine your cervix, we don't detect any significant change yet. I never tell women that they're in *false labor* though. I tell them instead that they're still in ripening phase. That just sounds more positive don't you think? And since keeping a positive outlook is so important as you prepare for labor, I like this better. No need to feel discouraged about contractions. No need to be disappointed that you've been contracting for a full 3 days and are still only 2cm! (This *is* normal). The contractions are doing something. They're getting your cervix *ready*.

How do we know the difference between ripening contractions and labor contractions? How many contractions does it take to get the cervix to dilate? Both good questions. You could have contractions on and off for hours or days during ripening phase. They start. They stop. They start again, getting you all excited; then fade away ... again. They tend to be mild and irregular. Of course it's hard to define "mild" because what's *mild* to one will be excruciating to another. You are all different. Typically "mild" means that you can politely answer a question during a contraction when asked.

Irregular is a little easier to define. You could have a flurry of contractions that come every 2 minutes for an hour, and then they go away. You could have contractions that come every 3 to 10 minutes for 14 hours, and then they disappear. What's a girl to do?? Ignore them! We'll talk more about strategies for coping with labor in Chapter Four. The simple answer for now is *try* not to make too much of them until they really grab your attention. And please—**don't** keep a record of them. They don't matter. We expect that you're uterus is going to contract. We want it to contract. What's more, it better contract or you're never going to have that baby!

The couples that make me smile are the ones who keep a contraction log. (Usually, only first-time couples do this. It's that bubbling enthusiasm that first time couples possess!)

I remember walking down the hall with one newly arrived couple asking "So, how far apart are your contractions?" The husband then whipped out his spiral notepad and began describing for me the sequencing of contractions over the past 3 days. I quickly rephrased my question to "So at what point did your contractions get to be consistently under 5 minutes apart?" The answer: 15 minutes ago. Without letting on, I guessed that unless they'd missed a few contractions, this lovely, enthusiastic client would soon be a disappointed couple. Another *in the door—out the door* first-time couple who needed some conversation about *fruit*—and ignoring contractions.

At some point though you'll want to get an idea how far apart contractions are. But wait till they feel like they're coming on top of each other to start timing. Please don't over analyze spacing. My Engineer clients really get into timing contractions. And moms tend to get very excited when contractions start because they think that contractions mean that the baby is on the way, and that's exciting! But contractions don't necessarily mean that the baby is on the way. They may just mean that your cervix is getting ready. Over focusing on contractions may set you up for disappointment—and we don't want you disappointed! We want you happy and relaxed as you approach your labor.

Contractions are timed from the start of one to the start of another. Now many women get hung up on the word "start" and can't quite figure out just when they started. It's ok. Time them from peak to peak then. Either way, it's a rough estimate. Our bigger question is "are the contractions doing the job?" Gross details about intervals and duration are somewhat irrelevant.

Since there's a huge emotional and psychological component to labor, you have to be careful about your focus on the contractions. The sooner you begin to focus on them, the higher your expectations become. The higher your expectations become, the more you set yourself up for disappointment if those contractions just aren't quite doing the job yet. So in truth, don't start timing them or journaling them until they begin to take your breath away. Up until that point, they're probably not doing more than ripening.

Here's the reason why timing early contractions can set you up for disappointment. The general rule of thumb today is that when your contractions are 5 minutes apart, lasting 60 seconds each, and they stay that way for at least an hour, it's time to go to the hospital. But based upon that advice, a lot of first-time moms won't be in labor. Many come to the hospital full of hope only to be told "I'm sorry Mrs. Jones; you're only in false labor. Come back when the contractions are closer." It's so discouraging because many of you will have been contracting like this for a long time and are still told "it's not time yet."

If you ignore them as long as possible rather than timing the early ones, it's more likely that you'll be pleasantly surprised when your provider examines you. But even if you're still not quite in labor yet, don't be discouraged. This is normal. All contractions are doing something positive for you—even the irregular ones.

Typically, contractions that do the job (i.e. cause progressive cervical change) are 2 to 3 minutes apart—for all women, even second and third time moms. If the cervix is good and ripe by the time contractions are coming 2 to 3 minutes apart it will usually dilate quite cooperatively. The rate of dilation will be different for everyone though (so don't compare yourself to your friends!) It doesn't matter what other women have done or what stories you've heard. Labor isn't a competition.

Women who've had more than one baby can dilate quite quickly if the cervix is ripe. But for first-time moms, 2 to 3 minute contractions will usually only make the cervix dilate about one centimeter an hour. Contractions that are farther apart than that will still be working on ripening.

I say this somewhat guardedly because I've seen just about everything. And I know that there are curve wreckers in every crowd! Knowing how your cervix is coming along in the ripening process may give you some idea how well it might respond when the contractions are finally perking along. So ask your provider for the details when he or she examines you.

In a nutshell, don't expect your cervix to dilate progressively until your contractions are 2 to 3 minutes apart. The first part of the process no matter how far apart your contractions are is ripening. (Are you getting tired of that word yet!) By that I mean *effacement*. Your cervix may dilate some in the early phases, but it won't dilate to big numbers until it's about 80% or 90% effaced. It all makes sense. It's harder to get the cervix to open when it's long and thick. Ultimately, all moms will get to the point where their cervix is 100% effaced and 100% open (or 10 centimeters) *if* they hope to have a vaginal birth. If they don't achieve this, they won't have a vaginal birth.

So if you come in for evaluation of labor and your cervix is 1 centimeter dilated and 50% effaced, I would think that you probably still have a ways to go. Especially if your contractions are only about 5 to 7 minutes apart. Of course there will be other things to consider before deciding whether to let you go home. But if the cervix is the deciding factor, then we'll probably all decide that being in your own home relaxing and resting is the best thing for you.

This question of "*am I in labor?*" really relates to the question that plagues every woman: "*Is it time to go to the hospital yet?*"

Most women want to go when they feel sure that they'll get their admission ticket and not get sent home. Lots of women worry about this. Let me just say to begin with that our doors are always open to you. It's ok to come and go home again—as many times as you want. Women do it all the time. We don't make you feel silly or stupid or even count the number of visits! We would much rather you come in and find out that everything is "ok" than have you at home brewing some sort of a problem. Most busy labor units see as many patients with questions each month as they do deliveries. It's normal, and I assure you that you won't be the only one.

Checking your cervix

Knowing whether or not you're in labor will require an examination of your cervix. Knowing how well your labor is progressing as you journey along will also require a cervical check. Knowing how the baby is coming into your pelvis is also determined by examining you internally. Your first exam will be around 38 or 39 weeks of pregnancy so that your doctor or midwife can see how ripening is coming along.

How do we do this? We do it with our fingers. We reach in (gently!) and try to locate the cervix. The cervix is found in the upper part of the vagina. In ripening phase, the cervix points toward your tailbone (called "posterior"). This means that when we reach in we don't find the opening right in front of us. Instead we have a bit of maneuvering to do in order to get our fingers around the corner and into the cervix. This is the only way that we can evaluate things like softness, effacement, dilation and station (how low the baby is). Checking the cervix—especially during ripening phase—can be a bit uncomfortable. But as the baby moves down and you move into labor your cervix rotates forward making it easier to get to.

What we're doing is creating a mental picture of what we feel. The whole purpose is to determine if the process is moving forward. When we check your cervix we know what's going on. We know if your cervix is ripening yet and how much ripening you're getting. We know if you're in labor and how quickly (or slowly) your labor is moving along. Each phase has its own unique qualities.

Another reason why your doctor or midwife checks your cervix around your due date is because it can help promote the ripening phase. Checking your cervix releases a little prostaglandin. Prostaglandin is a hormone that helps with ripening. So if that first exam is a little tough, remember that your provider is trying to do you a favor!

You can help make the exam easier by not fighting it. Easier said than done I realize, but the more you tense up and squeeze your knees together, the harder it is on your provider to evaluate your cervix. I know this doesn't sound very lady-like, but if you put your hands on your knees and pull them up toward your ears that posterior cervix becomes easier to reach and easier to reach means less discomfort for you!

When to go to the hospital

Since all you have to go by is contractions it can be confusing. If all is well with your pregnancy and your baby is moving, it's ok to labor at home for a while. It's nice to rest in your own bed and use your own bathroom. Some women worry that if they don't get to the hospital by a certain time they'll miss their opportunity for an epidural. The truth is that first labors are fairly long. Twelve hours on average—and that's *after* ripening phase. So you can see that there's a big window of opportunity for getting your epidural. Our hope—and yours—is that you just get there before the baby comes. (All the partners are nodding!)

Now I can't speak for every hospital when it comes to their epidural policy, but I think it's highly *unlikely* that you'll miss your opportunity. The reason is, again, that you have a pretty big window to work with. In general most hospitals are moving away from the number criteria—i.e. you can't have your epidural past 7 centimeters. This is because many first-time moms still have a lot of labor left after 7 centimeters, and it only takes about 30 minutes to place an epidural. Of course there are those who believe that if you've made it to 7 centimeters without an epidural you can make it all the way! This is true for most of you, but in 21st century North America we're pretty generous with anesthesia.

But the bottom line is, talk to your provider about his or her criteria for coming to the hospital. You might also want to get some information on the availability and philosophy of epidural services at the hospital where you'll be delivering. In general though you can expect your doctor or midwife to want you to come if:

- Contractions are strong and regular
- You have heavy bleeding
- Your baby isn't moving like normal
- You have weird pains in your tummy
- Your water starts leaking or gushing
- Or you're just not feeling well (headache, tummy pain, blurry vision …)
- And last, but not least, you can come whenever you want to! Our doors are always open to you. Even if you're not admitted, we'd rather you come and get checked out if you're not sure about something or have any concerns.

The downward journey

It's not often that we can say that something is 100% true for 100% of women. But when it comes to having a vaginal birth, we can. In order to have a vaginal birth, two things need to happen for all women: the cervix needs to dilate 100% of the way, and the baby needs to come down 100% of the way. If either process stalls and none of our tricks work to remedy the situation, then the baby is going to be born the *other way* (by cesarean section).

Even though it sounds a little scary, thank God for cesarean section! Women in past centuries and in many parts of the world have not had or don't have the blessing of cesarean birth available to them. Maternal and infant mortality rates demonstrate this. So if you're someone who thinks that cesarean birth is the worst thing that could possibly happen to you, please reconsider.

Before we switch gears though let's talk a little more about *descent*.

Descent is the process of the baby coming down and out. It all sounds so logical really, but when it plays out in real time it's not always so straight forward. It's amazing how tricky it can be to get these little people out!

I stumbled into a conversation about just this fact at a dinner party once. (Be careful inviting labor nurses to dinner parties!)

A friend was sharing her birth story and telling how the baby just wouldn't come down. She had labored a long time, but the baby was still very high. It was obvious from the telling that the whole process had been quite an ordeal for her and her husband. Both were still recovering from the shock of an unexpected cesarean birth.

After about 14 hours of labor her doctor examined her and found that not only was she finally 8 centimeters dilated (and 100% effaced), but the baby was coming down *face first*. This means that instead of the top of the head pushing into the pelvis and vagina, the baby was looking straight down the birth canal—nose leading the way. If you can picture this, you can imagine that this just isn't a good fit.

Before I could stop myself, out slipped a favorite quip. "Yep, it's sure a lot easier to get those little guys in than get them out!" The blank stares told me is was still too early for humor! (My intentions were good).

But the take away message is that *descent* can be tricky. You won't have much control over how the baby comes into your pelvis (or how big the baby is, or the size of your pelvis) ... This explains why you'll need to keep your heart and mind fixed on the things that really matter. Life is full of uncontrollable variables. And labor tops the list. If at the end of your journey you have a lovely healthy baby in your arms, that's all that really matters.

When it comes to descent, babies come into the pelvis in many differ-ent ways: bottom first, head first, feet first, arms first, or nose first. Most of these positions are automatic cesarean sections. The baby can't safely make the journey through the pelvis in some of these awkward ways. Head first is really the only way for most moms. But even in the head first position there are options.

If you picture your pelvis like the face of a clock, 12 o'clock being at the top and 6 o'clock at the bottom, babies can come down looking at any number. On top of that, some babies tilt their head sideways and try to give us their ear as a hand hold. Before the baby gets wedged too snugly in the pelvis he or she can turn its head. If the doctor or midwife finds the head is a bit cock-eyed, he or she might be able to turn the baby's head into a better position. And sometimes positioning mom can help turn the baby's head into a more desirable presentation, but sometimes nothing works.

The ideal head down position is called *occiput anterior (OA)*. This is where the back of the baby's head is up against your abdomen—in other words, the baby is looking down at your tailbone or hip. Take your hands and put them on your tummy, one on each side of your belly button. Now slide your hands down toward your groin and rest them there as you read the next sentence. Most babies will have the back of their head up against either your right hand or your left. This is called right occiput anterior (ROA) or left occiput anterior (LOA) respectively. Either one of these is the best fit through the pelvis.

If your baby comes into your pelvis looking *up* at your hands, this is called occiput posterior (OP) position. And this is not such a good fit through the pelvis. Now if you have a nice roomy pelvis and your baby isn't too big, vaginal birth is certainly possible. But many first-time moms wind up with cesarean sections because of the occiput posterior position. The fact that babies are also bigger these days contributes to the problem. One complicating factor can make vaginal delivery tricky; two can make it impossible. Big, "face-up" babies are tricky to get out.

In Chapter Five, "The baby in labor," we'll talk about how you might be able to coax the baby to turn into a good position. A baby in good position makes for an easier labor.

Let's talk about *station* now. Station is how we measure (with our fingers) how far down the baby is in the pelvis. We measure the downward movement of the baby's head in comparison to the bones of your pelvis. There are 7 stations that we describe and the distances between them are really small! Before the baby even comes into the region of "stations," he or she is floating in the uterus enjoying life in the hot tub!

As labor approaches your baby moves toward your pelvis. It's possible that your baby has been breech (bottom facing the door) your entire pregnancy and flips as labor approaches. It's also possible that your baby has gotten quite comfortable bottom down and won't want to move. Being able to turn depends on a variety of factors, like how wrapped up baby is in his or her umbilical cord or how bent or straight the legs are. Babies are quite flexible.

First babies tend to come into the pelvis earlier in pregnancy than second or third babies. If you're a first-time mom, you might notice that the baby seems to be dropping down around 38 weeks. People who know you well will notice that you're carrying the baby lower too. Of course sometimes people at the grocery store who don't know you at all notice too and make all sorts of comments that startle you! Be kind to them; they mean well. (I'm one of those people!)

There's a real advantage to the baby coming into the pelvis. For one, it gets the baby heading in the right direction. And two, if the baby comes down low enough it comes into contact with your cervix and helps stimulate the ripening process.

One of the obstetricians I work with describes this like pulling a turtleneck over your head. The more your head pushes into the "neck" the more the neck flattens out over your head. Women with low babies usually get really good effacement. And getting good effacement before labor starts often contributes to a nice short labor. This makes sense because effacement is such a lot of work. If much of it gets done before labor actually starts then the only process left to work on is dilation.

The unmentionables

Last but not least, let's talk for just a spell about the "unmentionables." These are the things that women want to know about, but are afraid to ask in polite company. So let's get them out in the open and clear away your fears. I don't want you to be worried about anything. It's all normal and we all know that labor can be a bit *messy*.

Mucus

It's no great mystery that women produce mucus, but when your body is getting ready for labor you'll produce *more* mucus. As your cervix begins to soften that overly popularized thing called a "mucus plug" begins to dissolve and come out. Sometimes the mucus plug comes out in one big blob while you're going to the bathroom, or it drizzles out slowly over time. It's nothing to get excited about. And it isn't necessarily a "sign" of labor. You could well have a week to go before labor starts after the mucus plug comes out. But it could be a sign that your cervix is getting ready—and that is exciting!

The mucus plug also has some old blood in it making it an unattractive shade of brown. As it dissolves the mucus discharge you get could be brownish in color. This isn't unusual. You may also have small amounts of reddish blood with the mucus as your contractions pick up. If you notice an unusual odor or bright red bleeding, you'll want to call your doctor or midwife and have it checked out.

Blood

Blood is another thing women are quite familiar with. One of the great joys of pregnancy though is that you *stop* bleeding on a regular basis—or you should. Spotting in early pregnancy is normal as the fetus implants into the rich lining of the uterus, but any other bleeding is considered abnormal and should be checked out. This isn't to say that bleeding during pregnancy means that the pregnancy is doomed, but it is cause for further investigation.

Bleeding typically comes from one of two sources: your cervix or your placenta. If you experience bleeding we'll want to make sure that all is well with your placenta. I really shouldn't say this, but I do want to help eliminate unnecessary fear: even if the bleeding is from your placenta, you'd be amazed by how much the placenta can bleed and still have enough power to support your baby.

The placenta is an amazing, resilient organ, **but at the same time** we want to be very certain that any bleeding from the placenta is *not* compromising the baby. So once again, if you experience any bleeding during pregnancy, call your doctor or midwife immediately and let them decipher whether there's reason for concern or not.

As your cervix begins ripening phase and moves toward labor, tiny blood vessels in the cervix open up and cause some bleeding. Another popular expression in this business is "bloody show" and this is what it means: that when you sit on the toilet and wipe you'll see bloody mucusy discharge. Truthfully, this is normal, but there's more to know. We'd want to know how far along you are (we don't want your cervix ripening before it's time), and if you feel the baby moving. Check with your provider and let them give you their answer to your symptoms. There may be something unique about your situation that needs more exploring.

Just so you know what to expect, many women see a lot of "bloody show" during labor. As your cervix opens and thins it bleeds. Quite often by the time a woman reaches 6 or 7 centimeters she's bleeding like a heavy period. It's not unusual, and some "bloody show" tells us that good things might be happening with your cervix. It's a sign that we watch out for as we evaluate how things are progressing.

Urine

Keeping your bladder empty during labor helps make room for baby. It's also true that sometimes during pushing phase urine comes squirting out with pushes. It's not unusual and nothing to be worried about.

Amniotic fluid

Once your bag of water pops a hole you'll leak amniotic fluid the rest of your labor. Often the baby's head acts like a plug and traps a lot of the water up around the body. When the baby's head jostles around though, more water will leak out. And it can be quite a lot! Every woman has a different amount of water, so you may want to wear a pad (or a towel!) when you're walking around or sitting in your favorite chair.

If you're positive for Group Beta Strep bacteria (GBS) your provider will want you to go to the hospital as soon as you can after your bag of water starts leaking. GBS can be harmful to the baby and standards of care dictate antibiotics be given to women with this bacteria to prevent infection in the baby. About 25% of women carry group beta strep bacteria. Your provider will test you for this somewhere between 36 and 37 weeks of pregnancy$_2$.

Passing stool

The thought of having a bowel movement during labor scares a lot of women. Please don't let it. It's all normal and doesn't bother any of us. Quite often your bowels will clear themselves during ripening phase as your body is getting ready for labor. But if you've had constipation problems and you're worried about this, give yourself a small enema at home or ask the nurse to do it for you. Unless you have something wrong with your bottom, this may help relieve your concerns about having a bowel movement.

Quiz

So let's have a little quiz and see how well I've taught you the definition of labor.

Which woman is in labor?

1. Mary is a first-time mom. Her cervix is 2cm dilated, 50% effaced, and her baby is at -1 station.

2. Delilah is a second-time mom and her cervix is 3cm dilated, 30% effaced and her baby is at -2 station.

3. Grace is a third-time mom. Her cervix is
1cm dialated, 100% effaced and her baby
is at zero station.

So who did you pick? Well, to be honest this was a trick quiz! If you said, "I need more information" you'd be right. If you're still locked into the idea that labor is a number, then you probably picked Delilah at a generous 3 centimeters. But the problem with Delilah's cervix is that it's still *really* thick at only 30% effaced and her baby is still pretty high.

Since Delilah has had a baby before, her cervix could well be 3 centimeters dilated just because she's had a baby before. Women who've had babies before tend to get some openness to their cervix without much effort long before they're actually in labor (lucky them!). But when Delilah's baby decides to come into the pelvis and push against that soft cervix, I would expect it to thin out nicely and dilate quickly. I would expect Delilah to have a nice easy labor once strong, regular contractions kick in.

Remember, labor is not a number; it's a rate of change. You don't have any information here about what these cervical exams were *yesterday* or even an hour ago. It's possible that all 3 are in labor and it's possible that none of them are in labor. We need more information!

If I had to pick the cervix I think most likely will respond to the power of contractions, it would be Mom Grace's at a mere 1cm. Why is that? Well, Grace has had 2 babies before (I'll add that both were vaginal births), so her cervix should respond well to the power of contractions. Also, she's already 100% effaced and that's a lot of work already accomplished.

The other thing that Grace has going for her is that her baby is quite low and obviously pushing hard into her cervix, that's why it's so thin. Also, second, third (and so on) babies tend to hang out a bit *higher* in the pelvis until labor really kicks in. So Grace's low baby tells me a lot! Like Grace is probably in labor and her baby is just about ready to be a newborn!

Of course, the last really important question to ask is *how far along these ladies are.* They'd all raise red flags if they were less than 36 weeks pregnant!

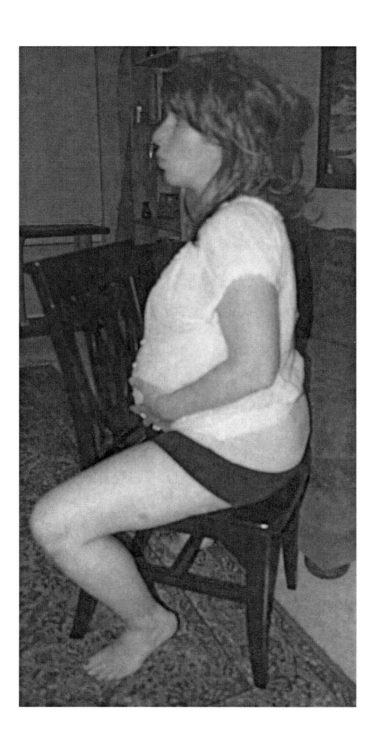

Chapter Two
Preparing yourself for labor

So before we start talking about birthing balls and bathtubs, we need to talk about something even more important: like what's happening in your mind.

Getting your mind ready for labor is probably more important than getting your body ready. And since you'll have more control over what happens in your mind than you will over what happens in your body, this is the right place to start.

This reminds me of a classic quote:

"Every action and feeling is preceded by a thought₃."

Where do our thoughts come from? How are your ideas about labor and birth evolving? You may be someone who's spent a lot of time thinking about your upcoming delivery, exploring every on-line conversation and interviewing all your friends. Or you might be one who prefers not to think much about it at all. There are women in every corner. Some want to know everything that they can get a hold of, and some don't want to know more than they have to.

It's said that knowledge is power, but I'm here to tell you that plenty of women have had wonderful deliveries and never cracked a book! Learning about the process and what to expect can certainly be helpful, but on the other hand over thinking it can work against you.

For the most part our ideas come from the influences around us and our interpretation of them. If we like what we hear (or see) we embrace it. If we don't, we reject it. For most of us, family members, friends, and media sources have the biggest influence over us and how we interpret life. Who are the most powerful people in your life? What are your most influential sources? And more importantly, how reliable are they?

Later in the book we'll talk more about the lively conversation taking place out in our world regarding the best way to have a baby. There are people out there with strong opinions! And I confess that I'm one of them. We all have our biases, typically developing from what we've seen and experienced. But sometimes biases develop based upon rumors and hearsay.

I want to encourage you throughout the rest of this chapter to examine your thoughts about labor and birth and consider where they're coming from. Are they fear driven? Are they inspired by someone else's story? How strongly do your hopes and dreams play into your decision making? Are you locked into a particular scenario? And if so, why?

The most important question though is *are your sources of information sound?* This last one's tricky, because we all want to believe that our sources are solid and reliable especially if we really like what they tell us. I don't want to discredit any of your favorite people, but I am asking that you think about the information that you're getting and begin to examine the thinking behind it. How you think affects the choices you make and not all choices are created equal.

A clear view of the goal

So for the purpose of exploring how your thoughts are developing, let's start with a little exercise. You'll have to humor me here because I won't be able to see if you're actually jotting ideas down, but it'll be so helpful for you as we journey through this topic to get some of your own ideas flowing.

I know that women talk to each other. We're relational beings, so of course we do! Brainstorm for me if you will the things that women have said to you about labor. Most women love talking about the day they gave birth and have all sorts of fun, interesting and dramatic stories to share. Jot down the some of the facts and figures that you've been given. What do they tell you? What have they said about labor?

Write your ideas in the box below.

So if your box is still blank go back and give it a try! Here's one to get you started: "My friend Sally told me she was in labor for 23 hours." What else have friends told you?

Pause for commercial break

I brainstorm this question with my prenatal classes and students (it takes them a while to get going too!) and the outcome is always the same. So I'm not expecting anything different from you. Here's how the list typically looks:

Women talk about:

- How long their labor lasted
- Where they delivered
- How much they enjoyed the bathtub
- That their bag of water broke at the grocery store
- That they finally got admitted to the hospital on their 3rd visit
- That they got induced a week after their due date
- How many hours they labored before they got their epidural
- What a wonderful coach their husband was
- How much they loved their nurse!
- That they were delivered by a midwife
- That the baby weighed in at a robust 9# 3oz.
- How sore their bottom was the next day
- Why they ended up with a cesarean section

And the list goes on …

Now, the next step in this *mindset* developing exercise is to see if we can come up with a heading for our list. What kind of a title would you give this list? What one or two words capture all of these comments?

Ok, I realize that I can only take this exercise so far without seeing you face to face, so let me just help you out with an answer!

Women talk about:

- How long their labor lasted
- Where they delivered
- How much they enjoyed the Jacuzzi tub
- That their bag of water broke at the grocery store
- That they finally got admitted to the hospital on the 3rd visit
- That they got induced a week after their due date
- How many hours they labored before they got their epidural
- What a wonderful coach their husband was
- How much they loved their nurse!
- That they were delivered by a midwife
- That the baby weighed in at a robust 9# 3oz.
- How sore their bottom was the next day
- Why they ended up with a cesarean section

And the list goes on …

Title: The EXPERIENCE of birth

When women talk to each other about their labor, the conversation usually focuses on the *experience* that they had: what they did, how everything went, what they wish had been different. Now am I setting you up to say that there's something wrong with this? No. But it's just not the *essential* focus. What is the essential focus? What is the most important thing about childbirth? What might be nice to mention when women talk about labor and birth scenarios with their expecting friends?

To answer this, take another look at this list and see if you can figure out what's missing. I tell you the truth when I say that this item is missing from *every* list that I've ever generated over the years with intelligent groups of people. And I'm actually not surprised. I'm not surprised because we live in the United States in the 21st century and we've gotten pretty good at things, so people don't see that it's missing. They tend to take it for granted even though they don't mean to.

Before I tell you the missing thing (though you may have guessed already), let me ask you another question. What's the *goal* of childbirth? Is the *experience* the goal? Let's add another dimension to our chart:

Women talk about: **The EXPERIENCE of birth** • How long their labor lasted • Where they delivered • How much they enjoyed the Jacuzzi tub • That their bag of water broke at the grocery store • That they finally got admitted to the hospital on the 3rd visit • That they got induced a week after their due date • How many hours they labored before they got their epidural • What a wonderful coach their husband was • How much they loved their nurse! • That they delivered by a midwife • That the baby weighed in at a robust 9# 3oz. • How sore their bottom was the next day • Why the ended up with a cesarean section • And the list goes on...	**The GOAL of birth:** Healthy baby Healthy mommy

Really it's a no brainer and I'm sure you all agree. It's so simple, why mention it? Well, there's more to it than meets the eye. We've gotten so good at the goal in 21st century North America that people tend to assume it. It's easy to take for granted that all will be well. This has led to a shifting in perspective toward *experience* being the primary goal (even though we know it's not).

It's the conversations that make me say this; conversations that I've had with many women and ones I read on the internet. Experience has become paramount. I'm concerned about how this shift in perspective is affecting women, from the decisions they're making about their birth experience to how they feel about it afterwards. If the experience doesn't play out as they hoped (at the hospital or in the home) many women feel devastated, even if they accomplished the goal.

This may not describe many of you who've given birth, but it does describe a growing number of women. Many women are nursing emotional wounds because they feel disappointment over the experience.

Those of us in the business don't take the goal for granted. We care about your experience, but we care about the goal more. I've had the privilege of experiencing birth in a number of places around the globe in some of the most *au natural* places imaginable, and perspectives are very different. Women who live in places where modern health care is virtually unattainable pray daily for the *goal*. They can tell you that the one and only important thing is a healthy baby and healthy mommy and they'd take whatever experience necessary to achieve it. Take a look at the following chart to get a feel for what I mean.

World Health Organization: Year of study 2008	
Maternal deaths for every 100,000 **live births** (that means that these numbers do *not* include moms who died if the baby died)	
Afghanistan	1400
Argentina	70
Bangladesh	340
Burundi	970
Congo	670
France	8
Indonesia	240
Israel	7
Laos	580
Mexico	85
Nigeria	840
Norway	7
Philippines	94
Somalia	1200
Switzerland	10
United States	24

Every number represents a life: a sister, a daughter, a mom, a wife. Raw numbers are interesting, but they don't tell the whole story. For one, it's really hard to collect perfectly accurate data which means that these numbers could be higher! Many people in the world live in really remote places and care providers may not have the ability or the motivation to report their tragedies. Cultural and societal taboos often lead people to keep things *hush-hush*.

Many things impact delivery outcomes, such as: What facilities and resources are available? What training is available to care providers (or *are* there care providers)? How similar are the moms in terms of age at delivery, number of children …? (Greater dissimilarity will lead to a wider range of issues.) All of these questions, and more, contribute to the numbers.

The point is that nowhere in the world have we arrived yet in our ability to protect every mom and every baby from the complications of pregnancy and birth.

Hospital birth has taken some criticism in the past decade. We've been told that we're "nervous" and overly attached to our devices and interventions. I might agree with some of the criticism to a point, but I see the full picture. What I also see is that some of the conversations out there present a limited view of reality. For no woman, no matter how well screened for potential risks is risk free. Every person in the business of childbirth knows that a *low risk* situation can become a *high risk* situation in the blink of an eye.

Health care providers are obsessed. I admit it. We are. And we should be. Labor and delivery is a tricky business. And sadly, we haven't perfected the process yet. Labor is unpredictable. The situation can change very quickly, quite often without warning, and none of us can see what the next minute holds.

Let me say again that we care about your experience *if* it contributes to the true goal and doesn't get in the way of it. For example, we won't wait for the cord to stop pulsating before cutting if the baby isn't breathing. Or we may need to cut an episiotomy if the baby's heart rate is dangerously low. You may have to trust that there are things that we understand in that critical moment that you don't and that all we want is the very best for you.

We most certainly want to help you have the labor of your dreams. But labor, like life, doesn't always go the way we want it to. Labor is fraught with uncontrollable variables. So if for some reason, your labor experience doesn't go the way you had hoped, please don't lose sight of what's most important.

We don't give grades or award trophies for birth. No one is keeping score. Without realizing it, some of the birth stories you hear can set you up for unspoken and unnecessary comparisons. For example, some women say things like "If Suzie can do it, I can do it!" Well, you may not have Suzie's hips! Women tend to compare themselves to everyone from the lady down the street with the fancy car, to some woman in some magazine with nice hair and stylish clothes. We want perfect fingernails, perfect bank accounts, and perfect kids. And we want the perfect birth.

Please don't compare yourself. Please don't set yourself up for disappointment by cultivating unrealistic and rigid expectations. (On top of that, if you're hoping for a natural childbirth, rigidity will be your biggest enemy!) Don't let anyone make you feel bad, inadequate, or like a failure as a woman if things don't go the way you hoped. You will do your best, and that's all you can you do.

I'm fussing over this because of how many grieving women I've cared for. Women who feel disappointed by any unexpected event or change in their plan. Women who weep because they delivered at the hospital instead of at the birth center, or who broke down and got an epidural, or ended up with a cesarean section. Of course grieving is natural when dreams are shattered. And with all the hormones floating through your system you hardly stand a chance!

But it brings great sorrow to my heart when I wipe tears from the cheeks of women who feel that somehow they failed. I admit that disappointment is painful, but no one should feel bad about their *experience* if that experience concludes with a gorgeous healthy baby nestled safely in their arms. Many haven't been so fortunate.

In conclusion, the experience of birth can be lovely and may go exactly like you hope. But it may *not* go exactly like you hope and you'll have no control over it. Even if we let the process go forward naturally, unmolested by modern medicine, things can go sideways. If we accomplish our goal of healthy baby healthy mommy we have cause for great celebration! Everything else is secondary. [If you're curious to know how you might respond if your experience doesn't go exactly as you hope it will, take the self-survey at the end of the book. Your results may give you some idea.]

A tale of two mommies

Once upon a time a mommy came to the labor unit to have a baby. She smiled cheerfully as I welcomed her to her room. She had that lovely first-time momma glow and enthusiasm about her. (I secretly hoped she was more than one centimeter!)

We had a nice time chatting and getting to know each other. She was very excited to be there and ready to try all the tricks and toys that she'd gathered. She told me that her due date was last week and that she had experienced a large gush of clear fluid 15 minutes ago, thus propelling her and her husband into the car and off to the hospital.

I knew by this report that Bonnie would likely get her "admission ticket," but labor seemed a ways off (I could tell by the smile).

I asked about her hopes for labor. Her husband then handed me their birth plan and explained that she was very committed to having a natural, non-medicated birth.

"That's great!" I said, "You can do it. Tell me a bit more about what that means to you."

When presented with such impassioned commitment to natural childbirth it means spending a bit more time gently exploring things. I needed to have some sense about their degree of commitment to this goal so I would know how to support them. Women often tell me they want natural childbirth and then follow up with the tag line "*unless it hurts too much.*"

Natural childbirth means different things to different people and I needed some sense of what was going on in her mind. More importantly I wanted to know what might happen if those things in her mind made a drastic change.

They told me that they had taken a great class on natural labor techniques and had been practicing together for the past month. Her husband then looked me in the eye and said quite assertively "I know my wife. And she wants natural labor." He didn't want any misunderstandings and I was now fully convinced.

Successfully reaching the goal of natural labor is usually a combination of factors, the *least* of which is a clever technique. The most important factor in achieving natural childbirth is plain, old fashioned determination (on the part of the client *and* the care giver I might add). Determination paired with an easy-going attitude is the best recipe for success.

When someone hands me a highly detailed, all CAPS birth plan, I see the determination factor, but begin to feel concern about the "easy going" factor. This then leads me to feel concern about the *disappointment* factor should we hit any bumps in the road.

After talking about some ideas and sharing with them my belief in their goal, I then asked my new couple, "So … how much would you like me to push you through the hard parts?" In the hospital setting, patients know that the candy man is just down the hall and I'm the mechanism for retrieving him. How will I know if she really wants to change her plan or if hints to that effect are just comments to be ignored?

Bonnie continued to leak clear fluid. An hour after arrival we checked and found her cervix to be 1cm dilated, 90% effaced and zero station. A nice place to start though Bonnie was somewhat disappointed. She had been 1cm at her last appointment and was hopeful that 5 days of random contractions had pushed her at least to 3. It wasn't easy to convince her that her cervix had ripened nicely and that all those contractions really had paid off.

So Bonnie and her husband decided to go for a walk. She had lots of energy and was ready to get the show on the road. About 3 hours later things began to pick up. She had been having 2 to 3 minute contractions since her arrival, but now they had her attention (the enthusiastic glow had lost some of its shine).

Bonnie was amazing. I was so impressed with her willingness to try new things, and her happy outlook between contractions. Her husband was the perfect labor coach. It was obvious that they had spent lots of time preparing for this special day. She tried new positions, rocked on the birthing ball, and took a shower. Her husband rubbed her neck and praised her after every contraction.

As time went on and things got more intense, we encouraged her to take a soak in the tub. She needed some relaxation. Even though the contractions were still 2 to 3 minutes apart, the warm bubbling water swirling around her helped take her mind off of them.

After another 4 hrs and lots of creative strategies, Bonnie appeared to be moving right along. She had come close to saying the "E" word several times, but her husband and I had successfully steered her in other directions. She rocked in the rocking chair, straddled the labor ball, and snuggled with her husband. At one point we encouraged her to crawl back into the tub on her knees where we showered her backside with nice warm water.

Labor nurses are pretty good at spotting waning determination. It's natural and happens to most everyone at some point. If one hasn't been through labor before, reality can be a bit shocking. And most typically that shock comes in the form of *time* and *intensity*.

Bonnie began to ask when her cervix would be fully dilated. I explained that everything was normal and that she was making good progress. She wasn't convinced but gathered her spirits and went for another walk.

Two hours later, Bonnie was exhausted—physically and emotionally. I could see that "I don't think I can do this anymore" look in her eyes. Once more I suggested that she crawl on the bed so her husband could put pressure on her low back. We covered the birthing ball with a fresh sheet and she rested herself over the top. She gently swayed her hips from side to side. After 5 minutes of this, she turned to her husband with tears in her eyes and whispered "I can't do this anymore."

When women reach that quitting point, I usually suggest checking the cervix. This can be another strategy for helping them get through a little longer. If I can eke things along to the pushing stage things usually get better. I really try *not* to check the cervix a lot because it can be discouraging to hear numbers that you don't want to hear—like 3 or 4. But, on the other hand, it can be *quite* encouraging to hear glorious numbers like 8 or 9!

I'd been waiting to see some of those lovely, telltale signs that Bonnie's cervix was completely dilated hoping beyond hope that she'd progress rapidly toward the pushing stage. Even though pushing is a lot of work the sensation is different and often more tolerable. But there had been no such signs, so I could only hope that she was at least 7 or 8 centimeters.

Bonnie was 7 centimeters 10 hours after checking in to the hospital. Even though this was great progress, Bonnie wasn't encouraged.

I discussed several more strategies with her and her husband including trying a small dose of medication. Sometimes a dose of IV medication can really help moms get some much needed rest and relaxation and get us more quickly to that desired pushing stage. I then said that I was going to let them have some private time to talk things over when her husband exclaimed "I know my wife, and she wants an epidural!"

I looked Bonnie in the eye and told her again what a good job she was doing, was she sure this is what she wanted? Did she want to try some medication? Did they want to have a few minutes to talk about it? She closed her eyes with tears on her cheeks and said "I really want an epidural."

Thirty minutes later Bonnie was resting comfortably in bed unaware of the contractions still coming 2 to 3 minutes apart. As I was fluffing pillows between her knees and arms I saw another large tear roll down her cheek. I brushed it away and put my hand on her forehead, moving hair out of her eyes. In a voice I could hardly hear she said "I'm such a wimp."

I looked her in the eye and replied "Do you tell your mom that she's a wimp when she wants Novocain for a root canal?"

"No" she smiled.

"Well, you are no wimp either. Labor pain is real. You've done an amazing job and should feel very proud of yourself. Don't you like your epidural?"

"I'm so happy! I haven't felt this good in weeks."

"Well, enjoy it then and be thankful you were born at this time and in this place! Try to get some rest now. Hopefully we'll be pushing very soon." I then sat down to do some much needed charting.

Almost immediately after this conversation, her husband left the room to get his bag out of the car. I followed him out the door to get some ice for Bonnie and saw that he'd been stopped by another couple just newly arrived on the unit. From the desk I could hear brief snippets of the conversation. I was *really* trying not to eavesdrop but I could see by his expression where the conversation was going. The new arrivals were friends from childbirth class and had just started into labor. In class, they had apparently made a pact, vowing to each other that nothing would deter them from a natural, non-medicated birth.

Rick was having a hard time confessing that Bonnie had just gotten an epidural. How I longed to step in, but I kept my peace. I hate to admit it, but I began praying fervently that this new couple would also succumb to the marvels of modern medicine! It was naughty I know for I truly did wish her every success. But I could already picture them bumping into each other the next day while strolling in the hall and my heart was heavy for Bonnie. It was already hard enough for her to accept that she had changed her plan. How was she going to face this friend the next day if that friend succeeded in having a natural labor where she had "failed"?

Why we women are like this, I don't know. We can be so competitive, secretly relishing any opportunity to boast about our accomplishments. But having a baby is no place for competition. Every happy healthy birth is cause for joy no matter how it's accomplished.

The next day I was dying to know how Bonnie was doing. I couldn't stand it any longer so took my lunch break to go knock on her door and say hello. I was so hoping that her remorse over having gotten an epidural had ceased and that she wasn't holed up in her room avoiding her friend like the plague.

I was delighted as I entered her room to see her and her friend holding their babies and laughing together. Both had gotten epidurals at 7cm and both were extremely thankful for them. What new joy they found together, both with gorgeous new babies and life changing stories to pass onto their friends. Without a doubt they both had bragging rights!

Preparing your body

Its common knowledge that second labors are about half the length of first labors. I suppose it makes sense if you think about it. If your body has been through the process before it has a better idea how to do it the next time. But the reason is even simpler than that. Once a body has been through the process things are more relaxed, meaning that the tissues give more easily the next time.

This truth defies one of the common myths about having a good birth: that a well conditioned body leads to an easier delivery. Now I'm not saying that it's ok to be out of shape! It's wonderful to be in good shape and you should take good care of yourself while you're pregnant. We're finding out more and more about how our entire life can be impacted by what happens during our time in the womb. For example, researchers are finding a link between how well mom eats and development of chronic diseases in her children later in life[5]. So please do try your best to be healthy and fit.

My point is *be reasonable.* Pregnancy isn't the time to start an enthusiastic exercise program. If you need to lose weight do so before you get pregnant. There is good research to show that being overweight increases your risk for cesarean section and other issues, so losing weight before you get pregnant is a good idea. Exercise is also a good idea. But choose something that won't traumatize your body, like walking or swimming. Talk to your doctor or midwife about what would be best for you.

Another simple idea for helping you prepare your body for labor is good posture. Most of you are too young to have had a grandmother who constantly reminded you to stand up straight! Good posture was a big deal to women of old, and maybe for more reasons than one. It may be that chronically poor posture encourages your baby to settle into the OP position[6]. Practicing good posture applies not only to walking but to sitting as well. The idea is to avoid slouching!

Gentle stretching may also help prepare your body for birth since giving birth is all about stretch. Loosening your limbs and increasing your flexibility, particularly the flexibility of your legs and hips might be very helpful to the process. Practice opening your legs and bending your knees, like when you sit on the toilet. If you're not used to it low squatting isn't a good idea. But placing your foot on a small stool or doing stairs are also good strategies for early labor. While you practice, think about relaxing all structures down there. This will be a good mindset for labor as it develops.

One last word of advice about preparing your body for labor. Rather than doing bottom tightening exercises, practice bottom rocking exercises. Pull your bottom forward and then let it relax. This may help your baby line up nicely with your pelvis. If you're a first-time mom you really don't need to have tighter bottom muscles; your bottom is tight enough I assure you! This is one reason why women having their second or third baby have an easier time—their bottoms give more easily. The right time to do bottom tightening exercises is *after* you deliver. We'll talk more about this in Chapter Seven.

Packing for the day

Pack light for your big day. In truth the hospital will have just about everything you need and it's nice to let them do the laundry! At the end of the book is a list with some ideas of things to take with you, but don't turn around if you forget something. Your husband or a friend can always go back and get things later.

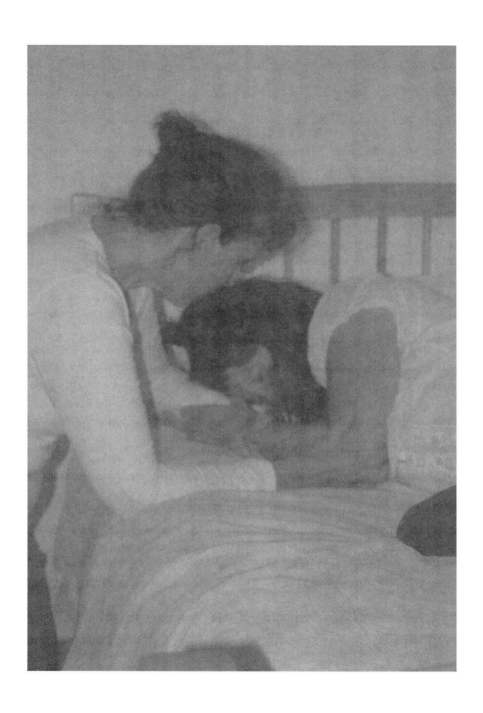

Chapter Three
Natural labor

Even if you plan to have an epidural, you can't skip this chapter! Because even if you plan on having an epidural you *will* experience some degree of natural labor before you're eligible for one. It might also be that you live in an area where anesthesia isn't readily available, or the anesthesiologist is not available at the *exact* moment you think you're ready. The bad news is that no hospital has an anesthesiologist waiting room (a room where they're just waiting for you to come). So gathering a few tricks might be very helpful.

Labor—with or without an epidural—is truly a wonderful amazing journey. Natural labor, by definition, it's delivering your baby without anesthesia. Some may also define it as delivering without any pain medication, but since we typically don't give medication within an hour of the anticipated birth, the actual *birth* will be fully non-medicated—thus, *au naturel*.

Women make the decision to pursue natural labor for many reasons. If you're really hoping for a natural labor, now's the time to do some soul searching and consider what may be motivating your pursuit. If you want natural labor because you think it's the best thing for you and your baby, then give it your very best effort. If your best friend had a natural labor and the two of you have been competing since childhood, this probably isn't the best motivation. It's really important that you come to the end of your journey **not** feeling that you're less of a woman if you change your mind.

Before we talk about tricks for helping you through natural labor (or any portion thereof), let's chat briefly about nurses and culture.

Some of you reading this book can't imagine anyone *not* wanting natural labor. And others can't imagine anyone wanting it. Sometimes these two groups of women have a really hard time understanding each other and it can be really tricky if your best friend falls in the alternative camp! Some women are fearful of birth because of all the stories they've heard, and some women live for a good challenge.

We who live in 21st century North America have it really good. We're blessed with conveniences and comforts unimaginable a century ago. In the realm of medicine, we're very thankful for all the solutions to so many of our problems, and living with *inconvenience* or *discomfort* is not part of our natural mental framework anymore.

The same thinking has come into health care and modern health care providers have very positive feelings about all they can offer clients these days. Especially when it comes to pain relief. We're very thankful for the ability to bring it under control or end it altogether.

Giving birth is painful (no matter what someone may have told you to the contrary). I don't mean to discourage you, but if you aren't realistic you'll have a hard time getting through.

Labor can also be painful for the doctor or nurse. Many care takers (midwives included) don't like to see their clients in pain, especially when they know that they can do something about it. You may think it odd for me to say that it's important that your care taker be good at natural labor if you desire natural labor, but it's true.

It's the belief that nurses and doctors are reluctant to support women desiring natural labor that's led some women to consider delivering in alternative settings. You make a pretty obvious commitment to natural labor if there isn't an anesthesiologist just down the hall for the nurse to call.

I'll confirm the truth of the rumor that some labor nurses aren't crazy about natural labor. Most labor nurses are infused with kindness genes. Truthfully, it's takes a certain degree of toughness to support women going through natural labor. Nurses are also taught that it's their job to alleviate pain, not support it. As a matter of fact, the organization that regulates and accredits hospitals instructs nurses to regularly assess pain and educate patients on pain management options. Thus most nurses are just hard-wired for pain relief.

For nurses supporting women pursuing a natural labor, the tricky part is knowing the difference between someone who really wants to persevere and someone who want to change their mind. It can be very hard to know the difference. If your nurse is less inclined to push you through the hard parts, any sign from you that says "I want to give up" will be enough for her to say the "E" word. Patients can be quite convincing when they say that they've had enough, but sometimes unfortunately we learn later that they really wanted us to ignore their pleas.

Labor nurses see this pattern on a fairly regular basis: mom who indicates that it's her desire to pursue a natural labor, who then changes her mind when things become tougher than expected. Unfortunately it's a pattern that has led a lot of nurses to doubt the seriousness of any stated desire for natural labor.

Since most moms want an epidural, your nurse will spend time trying to understand how committed you are to natural labor if this is your stated goal. This helps her know what her role looks like and how committed to natural labor *she'll* need to be when things get more intense. Of course if you come through the door at 7 centimeters with your wits about you she'll be fully convinced that you mean business!

Like anything, the more experience you have with something the better you are at it. At this particular time in U.S. history epidurals are still very popular and readily available. The point is that nurses who work in modern American hospitals have fewer opportunities to practice natural labor support skills and for some the intensity of natural labor makes them uncomfortable. Many are also more comfortable managing labor with an epidural in place because it allows them better control of the actual birth, giving the doctor or midwife plenty of time to get to you and deliver your baby.

The first step in being good at natural labor support is believing that epidurals are not necessary in order to have a baby because (in most cases), they're not. Again, it all starts with how we think. No one in the business (even those who prefer epidurals) believes that, under normal conditions, you *must* have an epidural in order to have your baby. We still acknowledge that they're a modern day luxury.

Having said that, there are times though when an epidural is an *excellent*, if not necessary, intervention. But since this is the chapter on natural labor, we'll talk about those things later.

Belief is a powerful entity. And in the pursuit of a natural labor, belief must come from both parties: the patient *and the provider*. It's as simple as knowing that you can do it: *because you can.*

So if natural labor is your goal, then the first step is to set your mind to it.

Spotting good candidates

Even though I believe that the vast majority of women can have a natural labor and delivery, some women are better candidates than others. It's true. Of course in the many years I've been laboring with women I've learned that nothing is written in stone. I'm surprised every day by what I see and experience. I think I have it all figured out, and kazam! The baby comes bursting forth in 2 hours instead of the expected 12. You have to love the unpredictable to survive this business!

But in general there are qualities or conditions that seem to favor the success of natural labor. When I first meet a new client I'm silently assessing her for these things, especially if she tells me that natural labor is her goal. It's important for me to know her for many reasons. One, it's my job to strategize care and anticipate where we're going (and how quickly!)

It's easy to know we're going to successfully have a natural birth if she shows up at 10 centimeters. (Women *rarely* come in at 10 centimeters so don't lose sleep over this!) It's not so easy though if she comes in at 2 centimeters completely exhausted having had contractions for 2 full days and then tells me she wants a natural labor.

Two, I feel a deep commitment to bringing my patient to the end of her journey getting as close to the experience of her dreams as possible. I don't want a sense of disappointment brewing in her heart as she looks in the eyes of her gorgeous new baby. It's worth saying again: the goal of labor is not the *experience*, it's the result—which is a healthy baby and a healthy mommy. So part of my assessment involves probing into her psyche to get a feel for what she really wants and how she might respond emotionally to a change of plans. Labor, like life, is an unpredictable journey and changing courses is normal. Some women accept this better than others.

So here are some qualities and conditions that seem to favor a successful natural labor:

Full commitment

Many women tell us they want natural labor. Some say this because even though they want an epidural, but they don't want it the second they hit the door: so "natural labor" *for a while* is their goal. Some want natural labor for every glorious moment of the journey and others, for some reason, feel obligated to try. Some women fear epidurals and others are morally opposed to them.

Can you see why we need to ask a lot of questions? It's important to sort the thinking out. But whatever the reason for seeking natural labor, the degree of commitment to this goal will be a key factor in successful completion.

Believe it or not, I hear this repeatedly from first-time moms when I ask their plan for labor: "I want to try to go natural—unless it's too painful." I give her credit for being honest since she's never been through the process before. But when I hear this I know that this woman will probably want an epidural sooner rather than later. And I won't be overly concerned because this statement reveals that she won't be.

The ones that are harder are the ones who seem very committed to the goal of natural labor but who have factors that might make the journey longer or harder. Labor in general is usually longer and harder than most women anticipate, but some variables make it even more challenging. For example, the persistently "sunny side up" baby (the "OP" baby) or when the water breaks before the cervix has done any ripening. Both of these conditions can make labor longer, and longer is harder.

Realistic ideas

Having realistic expectations will help you cope more effectively. The clash between reality and fantasy can set women up for unnecessary disappointment which is then counterproductive to the pursuit of a good experience. Isn't this true of life in general? Realistic expectations put us on the path toward peace and contentment. Fantasy sets us up for sorrow.

I've always said that it's better to come in with no ideas than too many. In this day of readily available information many women come in with strong opinions and resolute plans. Plenty of women never open a book or take a class and do just fine. Be realistic about your situation. Let go of unrealistic expectations. The easier you are on yourself, the better your body will respond to the process. The better your body responds the greater the chance you'll successfully accomplish the natural birth that you're hoping for.

Easy-goingness

Easy going, "go with the flow" women do better with natural labor (ask your family or friends how you rate in this department!)

When I meet a new client it's pretty easy to see if she's the easy going sort or more on the intense, controlling side of the equation. Since labor is unpredictable, having an open calm demeanor helps navigate the ups and downs of the journey. What's happening in your mind can have a significant impact on what's happening in your body.

We have a mischievous saying in Labor and Delivery (shared only amongst ourselves!) that the longer the birth plan, the higher the likelihood of a c-section. We don't mean to be unkind, but there's an important truth lurking in the humor. The woman who hands us an intensely detailed 10-page birth plan tends to be rigidly locked into a pre-set way of thinking. This often translates into rigid body parts and ineffective progress, making the journey long and grueling (for all of us!)

Ability to cope during the early phases

The woman who comes in repeatedly for labor evaluation during ripening phase is probably not a good candidate for natural labor. Of course, like I've said, anything is possible! Far be it from me to pre-judge anyone. But experience has shown me that if someone is having trouble coping in the early phases, she'll likely have more trouble when things get more exciting.

Most women consider that they're in labor when they hurt. Many women define labor as contractions. So it's a sad realization when they discover that pain and contractions don't necessarily mean that they're in labor. If their cervix isn't dilating yet it usually means that it will take *more* pain and *more* contractions to accomplish progressive change.

If I have a client who's intensely focused on her discomforts during ripening phase I suspect that real labor will be a challenge. If she's set on natural labor, sometimes a good heart-to-heart talk can help get this client focused. But if this is also the client who's given me that infamous 10-page birth plan saying that anything other than a natural labor is a failed experience, I'm worried. For not only is she likely to change her mind, she's going to be seriously disappointed about it.

Generous admitting exam

Being "admitted" to the hospital changes expectations, and when your expectations change, so does your focus. Expectations are so powerful. When you get admitted you feel, and rightly so, that we've declared to you that you're in labor. But the truth is that many women get admitted to the hospital when they're still in ripening phase.

How does this happen? Well, for one the transition from ripening phase to labor phase can be very subtle and the person making the decision *suspects* rather than *knows* that you're in labor. If you're a bit on the theatrical side, you'll be more likely to get your admission ticket—but don't assume that you're in full-blown labor. Full-blown labor may still be down the road.

When we make the decision to admit you we do so by gathering a large amount of information, and then make an educated guess. Sometimes we don't need to wait to see if your cervix is actually *progressing* before we make the decision to admit you because it's obvious. You're 5 centimeters dilated, contracting every 2 minutes and hysterical. At other times it's not so obvious. The decision is made to admit you because all the factors *seem* favorable (i.e. the cervix is well effaced, contractions are regular, and you're struggling with the pain).

The point is, if you get admitted at 1 centimeter and spend 99% of your labor at the hospital, it will set you up for expectations that'll make it harder to accomplish a natural labor. This is because women who are at the hospital a long time become intensely focused on every tingle and twinge. This scenario opposes the number one strategy for successfully accomplishing a natural labor which is to *not* focus on your labor. Women admitted in very early labor or, God forbid, ripening phase, are less likely to successfully accomplish a natural labor.

Is it "bad" to be admitted early in the process? No, but if everything is normal it's better to be at home. The problem is that most hospitals don't have the luxury of having women percolate in a *non-admitted* capacity for hours. When you're there we're responsible for you. We need to take care of you—by law. So if you are still deep in ripening phase, thinking that you are in labor (but going nowhere fast), the temptation to "help" begins to loom large. We wish we could let you do your 54 hours of remaining ripening phase and 12 hours of labor phase at the hospital, but that just isn't going to happen. Words like "oxytocin" and "break your water" begin to get passed around.

Thus, it's more likely that you'll successfully accomplish a natural labor if you show up in well established labor with your cervix nicely dilated to something other than 1, 2, or 3. (Seven is a nice number!) Just as long as you show up before the baby does!

Steady or rapid progression

Obviously, a shorter labor is easier to accomplish naturally than a long one. It doesn't mean that a short labor is an easy one, but it is "easier" to feel pain for 2 hours rather than 10. Though of course we only know the length of labor in hindsight, and no one feels their labor is *short* when they're in the midst of it.

This is the problem. No one knows where the finish line is until we're there. As care givers we can offer an educated guess, but labor can be very surprising. It's happened to me many times that I predict a long labor, and it's short. Or I predict a short labor, and it's long. We really can't know. It would be so helpful in your pursuit of a natural labor if I could say "Your baby will be here at 4:52." This would give you a clear goal to shoot for and peace of mind knowing that the pain will come to an end at 4:52. But alas, life isn't like that (nor is having a baby).

One day a woman came bursting through the doors crying at the top of her lungs. We knew instantly that something was up! It was her second baby and her cervix was 8 centimeters dilated with a bulging bag of water pushing through. (This means that the baby was pushing down hard and the bag was ready to burst).

She was desperate for an epidural. Between coaching and preparing for the birth, I calmly assured her that we were doing everything possible to get her ready.

As others set a delivery table and got warm blankets, I listened to the baby's heart beat and helped my new patient with her breathing. She begged me again for something to take the pain away and I calmly assured her (again) that we were getting ready as quickly as possible. (I wasn't lying. We were getting ready as quickly as possible, but not for the epidural. We knew what she was soon to find out. Her baby would be here long before the man with the needle. No need to add sorrow to suffering though!)

With the next contraction her water broke spraying amniotic fluid over the bed and onto the floor. I moved to the foot of the bed and lifted the sheet. Quietly I said "give me a little push."

It was at that moment that she realized, to her horror, that the epidural man was not coming her way. But the overwhelming urge to push tore every other thought from her mind.

Just as the doctor donned his gloves she gave two powerful pushes. Out came her baby and into her arms. It never entered her mind that she could do it, but she did. And she was delighted! The whole experience took only 5 minutes. This was natural labor at its best!

Labor can take a direct route or a circuitous route. Anything is possible when it comes to dilation or descent. In general, the cervix dilates about 1 centimeter an hour when you're in active labor. Once your cervix starts making progressive change it can scoot along quite quickly *or* it can stall for a spell.

This is can be frustrating for the woman hoping for natural labor. To help avoid unnecessary mental anguish, I try to examine the cervix only when I think I have good news to report. Even so, if the number you hear is *less* than the number you hope to hear it can cause your countenance to fall. The truth is that labor will proceed at its own unique pace.

It's easier to accomplish a natural labor if things progress quickly and in a straightforward manner. If it doesn't, it can be hard to push through. This is where a committed caretaker comes into play; otherwise he or she may be the first to say the "E" word.

Watching you struggle while getting nowhere could be just the opportunity they need to suggest a new plan. It takes a care provider who can wisely discern the difference between truly *stuck* or a bump in the road to help guide the way. The only thing that will tell anyone the difference between the two is **time**. And during this time it will take lots of mental and emotional support along with some creative thinking to help get you through.

If time reveals that you are truly stuck, then the relaxation that you get from an epidural could be exactly what it takes to help you get over the bump.

Good hips

Have you ever heard the *Beefalo* story? Once upon a time, North American cattle ranchers decided to develop a new product—beefalo. As indicated, this new creation results from crossing cows and buffaloes.

It sounded like a great idea, but they ran into some problems. Big daddy buffalo crossed with small mommy cow led small mommy cow into some tricky territory. Ultimately they found that it worked better when they bred daddy bull on mommy buffalo.[7]. I suspect it had something to do with pairing the right size baby with the right size hips!

The moral of the story is if daddy is twice your size, you may run into trouble too! If your baby is an easy fit through your pelvis, the easier your labor is likely to be. We're always on the lookout for these kinds of things.

There's an old wives tale out there that says that the size of your pelvis is related to the size of your shoe. So if you've been blessed with big feet (but always longed for size 6 petites) now's the time to be thankful!

It seems to be that tall, normal weight women have an easier time delivering large babies than short women. So it may be that there's some truth to this tale after all, for tall women usually have bigger feet too. But, the bottom line is we really can't know how big of a baby any woman can deliver until we try.

Since getting through labor naturally is 90% mental and 10% "tricks," we've spent this time talking about insights from the realm of the mind and exploring good candidates. But tricks can be helpful too! The next chapter takes us deeper into the nitty-gritty of getting through labor and offers more ideas for helping you maneuver the challenges both mentally and physically.

Whether you hope for a natural labor or plan to have an epidural, the following strategies can help you through your journey and make it the best of all experiences!

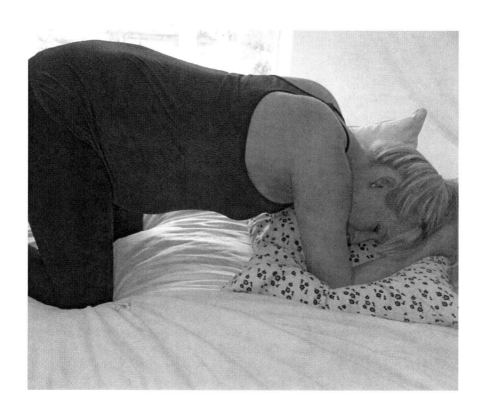

Chapter Four
Strategies for coping with labor

This is where the rubber meets the road! And this is where a good labor coach is worth their weight in gold. No matter your plan for labor you'll need a few tricks for navigating the journey. Don't worry about trying to memorize them all though because your nurse or midwife will help you through.

Determination and belief
We've already talked about the fact that old-fashioned determination is essential if you want a natural labor. It will also take some fortitude even if you plan to have an epidural, because—well there are no guarantees! Even if you do get an epidural you'll have some work to do before you're eligible.

Women are amazingly strong. And most are stronger than they think they are! You need to do some positive self-talk and tell yourself that you can do this—because you can. The road before you has been paved by many a brave soul. Let them inspire you!

Underestimate what's happening
Focus is everything. We talked briefly about the fact that once you're admitted to the hospital your focus will naturally shift to the *process*; to what's happening *in* and *to* your body. While this is understandable, it's not overly helpful. I can only speak for myself, but we women can be quite self-absorbed. Putting ourselves on center stage comes very naturally for many of us (especially first-borns like me!) When you're in labor you expect, naturally, to be the center of everyone's attention.

The problem with this is that it gets you all excited about things that you really shouldn't get excited about. Of course it's exciting when signs of labor begin. But signs of labor can start showing up a week before actual labor starts. If you start fixating on every tingle and twinge at the very start of the process it's going to be a *very* long journey for you. The woman who does this makes 5 trips to the hospital before true labor starts and feels completely defeated and demoralized by the time she's 2 centimeters. Feeling discouraged before labor actually starts will make it harder for you to weather the ups and downs of the journey.

This is what happens to women who are given their admission ticket in ripening phase or very early labor. I see them "monitor watching," saying things like "Oh honey, look at that one! That one hit 80!" (All the while she's smiling and laughing.) What this woman doesn't know is that we're not watching the monitor; we're watching her face! If she's smiling and laughing the contraction isn't doing much, even if it hits "80." [The monitor paper shows contractions as humps. Small humps register somewhere between 30 and 40, and big humps register between 70 and 100. Clients often believe that the size of the hump reflects the strength of the contraction, but this isn't true. Since the monitor piece sitting on the skin can't measure intensity, the size of the hump is actually irrelevant. We really aren't watching the size of the humps to tell us how strong the contractions are anyway. What we're really watching for is how the baby copes with contractions when they happen. So any size hump will serve the purpose.]

And that's because the monitor isn't measuring the strength of the contraction or its effectiveness. *It's only sensing a change in muscle tone.*

This focus on the process gets many women all keyed up. And being keyed up leads to tension, and tension hinders the process. Thus, one of the most important strategies for coping with labor is to **underestimate**, rather than overestimate, what's happening. Forget it. Don't pay attention to the monitor or the contractions. When labor means business, you'll know it. Until then, don't think about it.

Don't focus on the contractions
I'm going to say the same thing again, but in a slightly different way so it really sinks in.

You have to have contractions, and you have to have a lot of them. One contraction means nothing. Your uterus is a muscle and muscles contract. The best strategy for getting through labor is to ignore them as long as possible. Don't stand around your house and say things to yourself like "Was that one? I think that was one." When they're doing their job you won't need to guess.

I know I'm going to get myself in trouble with the techy world, but please don't use your cell phone to keep track of contractions. We don't care how many contractions you've had or exactly how far apart they are. We just want a rough idea. We know when we see you how the contractions are doing.

Here's an inside secret for you. When you come in, we begin running some unspoken visual and tactile tests on you. Your face is our first study. It tells us a lot about the effectiveness of the contractions. Some women though are on the, shall we say, dramatic side. So when I'm not certain about what my client's face is telling me, I purposely wait for a good contraction to hit and then calmly ask a question. Right in the middle of it! If you're able to politely answer my question, I begin to suspect that you're still in the early phases. Ultimately, though, your cervix will be the judge.

The best strategy is to let the contractions come and let them go. Don't comment on them; don't worry about the next one. Focus on the lovely breaks that you get between them. And this is our next helpful strategy.

Focus on the rest periods

This is the big one. This is an ***essential*** strategy if you hope to successfully accomplish a natural labor. You must have the right focus—and the contraction is not it. Of course it can be very hard *not* to focus on the contraction, but do the best you can. I tell clients that the contraction only lasts 60 seconds. And you can do anything for 60 seconds, right? Let contractions come, and let them go.

The focus of your labor needs to be on the wonderful rest periods that you get *between* contractions. Now granted, the rest periods not very long, but they're *very* important. This is where you rest and re-energize. I frequently remind my clients to soak up the rest period. I point out to them that the contraction is fading away and help them gear down for their next wonderful break.

When things are intense they often don't realize that the contraction is fading. Telling them that it is gives them hope that the rest period is right around the corner. "It's coming down. Now rest. Rest." Let everything slide down: shoulders, arms, tension. And rest.

As labor progresses, you may not feel that you're getting a rest period. It can feel like you're contracting all the time. What happens in labor is that you begin to feel more of the contraction. Contractions don't necessarily get closer in active labor, but you feel the contraction from beginning to end. Since contractions in real labor come about every 2 to 3 minutes, the rest periods don't seem very long, but they're critical. Develop the habit of soaking them up.

This is where your support people can really help you. They can see the tension in your body and shoulders and help you do your best to let it go as the contraction fades away.

Don't leave home too soon

Everyone wants to know when it's time to go to the hospital. The correct answer is "anytime you want to." Our doors are always open to you. We'd rather you come in and discover that everything is ok, than have you stewing at home brewing a problem. *It's not a crime to get sent home.*

If all is normal a good rule of thumb is to come when contractions mean business. But if you want to be as sure as possible that they'll give you your admission ticket, or you want a natural labor, don't go to the hospital too early. Wait until the contractions are consistently at least 3 minutes apart.

For the vast majority of women the cervix won't dilate progressively until the contractions are at least 3 minutes apart. Based on the 5-1-1 rule (one hour of contractions—5 minutes apart—that last for one minute), most first-time moms won't be in labor yet. It's the rare woman who will actually dilate at any sort of progressive rate with contractions no closer than 5 minutes apart.

It's also nicer to be at home! You can eat ice cream and wear your cozy pajamas. Once you get to the hospital you'll be relegated to popsicles

and shapeless gowns. (You'll certainly be able to wear your favorite pajamas in the hospital too, but you probably won't want to take them home
afterwards.)

Go with the flow

We've talked about this a bit already, but it's worth saying again. Letting
yourself go will help you dilate. Of course when you hurt it's easy to tense
up and squeeze body parts, so you can only do your best. Here's a visual
for you to think on. Picture floating in one of those little rubber rafts on a
river. Rather than trying to fight your way upstream, picture sinking into
the raft and let yourself float downstream.

Distraction

This makes sense. If you aren't supposed to think about yourself, your
contractions or the process, what are you supposed to think about? The
answer: anything that makes you happy! Many women find it helpful to
have a focal point completely unrelated to what's going on around them.

I once attended the birth of a very dear friend. She kept her eyes
glued to a goofy card I bought with a baby hanging in big underwear from
a clothes line that read "Hang in there baby!" I didn't buy the card for that
purpose, but for some quirky reason she found this to be her most helpful
focal point.

It's also really important for you to come out of your contraction and
look at the world around you. Smile. Be happy. Relax. As labor progresses
it'll get harder to do this. But, the longer you can keep a happy heart the
better your chances of getting through without medication.

Keep your heart light

You are all different and the circumstances surrounding your labor will
be unique to you. I don't want to assume that each one of you reading
this book is facing labor with a happy heart. It may be that your partner
is deployed overseas or that your baby is coming into the world with a
known challenge. I've seen the hard side of life too and don't mean to

trivialize your situation if this is your story. But for most women, trying to keep a light heart will help get you through the process.

By keeping a light heart I mean that you keep from getting too worked up over inconsequential things. Like the fact that your husband forgot to pack your favorite nightgown, or that your labor started before you finished childbirth classes. So many things won't matter 20 years from now!

Try to keep a sense of humor

This is something you'll need for parenthood too, so no better time than labor to start practicing!

(Warning to loved ones: humor is a great distraction strategy, but as labor progresses the ability to appreciate humor vanishes. Give it a try while you can, but lock it away when you see her smile disappear.)

We never know where the finish line is

The hard part about labor, besides the fact that it hurts, is that you never know when the hurting will come to an end. In retrospect, many women will say "I could have done it if I had known it would only be that long." Yes, if we knew many of the things beforehand that we know now, how different life would be! But where would the fun be? The mysteries of life are what make the journey interesting.

The best way to deal with this challenge is to take it one step at a time. Just do the next thing and try not to think too far down the road. The good news is that I've never met a woman who was pregnant forever yet. You will come to the end. You will have a point of delivery. I promise.

Have your cervix checked only on a "need to know" basis

In truth you may not have much control over this one. I'd like to believe that care providers only check the cervix on a "need to know" basis. But the truth is that we tend to be a little obsessive-compulsive about what's happening in there. There are times when we need to know, but my personal belief is that those times occur a lot less frequently than we think.

I'd love it if we only checked the cervix twice: once on admit, and once to say, "You're complete! You can start pushing now!" (A collective gasp of disapproval just filtered through the obstetric community). But, as idealistic as I am I realize that this is just a pipe dream. Life isn't so simple.

Our obsession with checking your cervix relates to the reality that when you get admitted we have expectations for your progress (this is one of the complaints against hospital birth). When you get admitted we expect you to progress at a reasonable rate, and in order to know if you're progressing at our expected "reasonable" rate we need to check your cervix. (Another inside secret: there are a variety of opinions out there on what "reasonable rate" means. Rate of progression can be really variable between women and all care providers have different expectations.)

But if you're trying to accomplish a natural labor, it can be so discouraging to hear how far you have left to go (or so it may seem). This is why I need a better reason than pure curiosity to check a cervix. Again, labor can do just about anything. Some women (especially second, third, etc time moms) can dilate quite quickly after 5 centimeters if their cervix is soft and stretchy. But first-time moms tend to stick more closely to the "one centimeter per hour" trajectory.

I also try to avoid the question *how far dilated am I?* as long as possible because of how the answer may impact my client's psyche. The number is basically irrelevant anyway. The baby is here when it's here. If he or she isn't here yet, we keep working; one step at a time, one contraction at a time. Soaking up the rest periods every chance we get.

But when all my tricks seem to have lost their charm, and I sense waning enthusiasm, I may suggest checking the cervix for the purpose of inspiring motivation. The hope being that when I check the cervix the number we discover serves to inspire my client onward rather than prompting her to give up. It may also be that I can give her some sort of time frame to work with and encourage her to believe that she's nearly there.

So you see, the knowledge of how far dilated you are can either encourage you or discourage you. The bottom line is, try to not think about. Just tell yourself that the baby is coming, and will most certainly come in due time.

That should give you a few more **psychological**
stratagies to work with.
Let's talk now about some **physical** strategies that might
help you in your journey through labor.

Relaxation

Many of our tricks and strategies are designed to help promote relaxation because, without a doubt, relaxation helps move the process forward. Relaxation also does wonders for your countenance! If you feel more relaxed, even though you're having pain, you may well feel that you can cope better with it and keep taking the next step forward$_8$.

In some way every new fangled (non-medical) idea for managing pain is really just a new twist on relaxation. Helping women get through natural labor or any portion of labor naturally requires some creativity (and psychology). It's not that anyone has the be-all and end-all trick [When you're exploring your options it's important to remember that some people advertise things that seem to make sense, but haven't been proven. It's good to try new things, but childbirth is no place to experiment with untested and unsupported practices. Every provider, whether in the hospital or in the home is promoting a business]; we're all just trying to help you get down the road. It could be that any number of tricks will make you feel better and move the process forward. It could also be that standing in one position swaying side to side your entire labor will be just as effective.

Sometimes tricks are about moving things forward (physically), but more often they're about keeping *you* moving forward (mentally). I say this because you'll hear some women swear by some particular trick or strategy that they feel "worked" for them and you won't like it. Or you find that it doesn't help your labor move forward. Don't let this discourage you. Every woman has a different set of variables and what one person likes isn't necessarily what someone else will like.

Maybe the trick really did push labor forward or turn the baby or shorten the pushing stage. But maybe the trick's most powerful impact was *mental* not *physical*. Maybe things would have gone just as well with another trick or without any tricks.

Your mental state is critical in labor, so if the trick makes you feel better and helps you cope, that's great. On the other hand, your provider will help you know if maybe you need to consider a new trick because things *aren't* moving forward physically with that particular trick. Your mental state is important, but ultimately it's the physical that matters (i.e. having the baby come out!)

Be open to moving around

I have different recommendations for this strategy based on where you're at in the process. In the early phases we tend to make you walk until you have blisters on your feet, mostly because we're all so anxious to get the show on the road. But walking in *ripening phase* will not put you into labor. Walking in *early labor* may stimulate more discomfort, but it won't necessarily make the contractions more effective. When hormone levels build up, so will more effective contractions.

The truth is labor can start while you're sleeping. And too much walking has a down side: strained ligaments, sore legs, painful feet, and achy back.

> **Ripening phase is the time to just live your normal life.**
> **Early labor phase is the time to rest and**
> **do whatever makes you happy.**

Once you're in solid labor (your cervix is making progressive change) it's important to move around and fight the urge to become catatonic (i.e. finding one position you like and never moving from it). Many women move around naturally; others need some coaxing. Moving and changing positions can help the baby find a good path through your pelvis. The baby has several maneuvers to make as it journeys from your uterus to the outside world, and keeping your hips and pelvis loose and relaxed can help baby navigate the corners[9].

Try something new about every 20 or 30 minutes; even if the new thing is as simple as putting one foot on a small stool, or bending over rather than standing upright. There are lots of different positions you could try or things you could do. Your caretakers will have their own favorite tricks and will help you explore ones that might be best for you.

The point is, *be open minded and give them a try* even if you're planning an epidural. We never know which small movement might help move things forward. We do know though that moving around can do wonders for your frame of mind!

Here are some ideas to try (barring any known objections):

- Kneel on the bed and swing your bum from side to side
- Lean over the bed and rock your bottom back to front
- Climb some stairs sideways
- Turn from your left side to your right side when you're in bed
- Bend your knees while you're walking
- Rearrange your legs every so often
- Rock in the rocking chair with a pillow behind your back
- Sit on the birthing ball
- Lean over the back of the bed
- Straddle a chair
- Sit on the toilet
- Dangle from the squatting bar
- Dance with your partner

Stay loose

Loose is just what it sounds like: *loose*: hands, neck, back, and hips. Dangle your arms, sway your hips and swing your bum. As things move along and things get more intense staying loose is tough. Even if it's hard to stay loose during the contraction, get loose during that wonderful rest period. I'm convinced that the stalls that we often run into during labor happen because of increasing tension and rigidity. This is why laboring in the tub is so wonderful. Warm, soothing water swirling around your body is a fabulous way to help promote relaxation. (But that's coming!)

Good breathing

If your contractions aren't doing something to your breathing (like taking your breath away) they're probably having minimal effect on your cervix.

That's why we ask you a question at the peak; because we're trying to figure out if it's the real thing or not. If you're body isn't forcing you to do some odd breathing during contractions then we suspect that it may be because the cervix isn't responding much yet. (I don't mean to discourage you, but being realistic is important so that you *don't* get discouraged.)

Good breathing is critical. It's good breathing that will help you stay loose, or as loose as possible. (If you're 8cm and going natural, you're not going to be "loose" during contractions. But, you can get loose during the rest periods with good breathing). Quite often women need a good coach to help with breathing, someone they can't overpower or ignore. This is when a good nurse or doula is worth every penny. No hard feelings later!

Good breathing helps you keep your wits about you and stay focused. In the early stages of labor you should be able to do slow *blowing* type breathing, like you're *slowly* and assertively blowing out a candle. With each slow outward breath let your shoulders fall. This is the important part because it's not the breathing per se that's helpful. What you're really shooting for is the relaxation that the breathing facilitates.

It doesn't matter if you breathe in through your nose or your mouth, though I think it's easier to breathe in through your mouth. When you breathe out though, you most definitely want to do so through your mouth. Pucker up your lips and blow out hard letting all the tension go. Listen to the breath coming out of your mouth. Listen to it. Focus on the sound of it. This is a *good* focal point. And let yourself melt. Then as you come to that lovely rest period, you're ready for it. Practice this at home.

This is really all there is to it. I encourage clients to stay with this hard-blowing, tension-releasing sort of breathing until it's obvious that we need a change in strategy. The next strategy is necessary when loss of control is brewing. So, hopefully if you're trying for a natural birth, you're a ways down the road when this switch in strategies is necessary. If you plan on having an epidural you probably won't ever need to use this next strategy.

The other breathing strategy is patterned breathing. Practicing this before you're in labor can feel a bit silly, but in order to get through the latter parts of labor you'll need a good patterned breathing strategy. You've probably seen a unique variety of patterned breathing techniques demonstrated on your favorite sitcom, so pick the one you like. Like "Hee, hee,

hee, hoo" (or "Waa, waa, waa, woo!") It really doesn't matter which one you use, it's more important that you stick with it.

I've seen some of the most amazing and effective patterned breathing techniques that women have crafted themselves. One woman had practiced a very unique—and effective—counting technique ahead of time with her friend. The friend said a number and the woman panted that many times. The friend was always a step ahead, sitting face to face leading the way from the beginning of the contraction until its glorious conclusion. It was like watching art in motion.

Many clients come in without a favorite, so I teach them mine. Simply blow 3 short, one long "**pu**," like "put" without the t on it. You sort of say it and blow it at the same time, "pu, pu, pu, puuuuu."

Most women need help staying with patterned breathing during those powerful, late stage contractions. When I'm coaching a woman in late labor I get about 12 inches from her face during the contraction, put my finger between us and ask her to blow on it with me. It takes a lot of focus and a lot of determination to push through this stage. But you can do it. We're all here to help you and we believe in you!

One last word about breathing. It's easy to hyperventilate in labor. This is when you're breathing so fast that you really aren't breathing effectively! This type of breathing can make you feel dizzy, light headed and tingly. It's also not good for the baby Over time, breathing too fast can hinder oxygen flow to the baby[10]. So if your hands or mouth begin to feel tingly, hold your breath for a few seconds between contractions to help reverse the situation.

My patient Carrie was deaf and really wanted a natural childbirth.

Her doula Sarina signed and was determined to help get her there.

I confess that I felt bad that I couldn't offer more in the coaching department, but what I witnessed that day is memorialized in my mind forever.

The two of them worked as one unit—face to face, giving and responding. Carrie tried a lot tricks in the early phases, but as she pushed closer to 10cm Sarina got closer, inches from her face, commanding her attention.

Carrie fought the urge to close her eyes and disappear into her own private world of pain, but she willed her eyes to follow. Sarina's fingers never left Carrie's face. She brushed her cheeks with her fingers, forcing her to follow her lead and stay with her breathing. Contraction after contraction, hour after hour they climbed the mountain together, each flushed pink and glowing.

Eight hours and 22 minutes later, Carrie gave birth to her second gorgeous son.

I'd never felt so honored to have such a job.

Be open to the tub or shower

The tub is a wonderful place to spend some time! Some women though are shy about trying the tub or the shower. I'm not sure if it's the getting naked part or the getting wet part, but whatever part might hold you back try to overcome it. Give it a try, even if it's just for one contraction. It might be that once you discover how lovely it is, you won't want to get out! And remember, relaxation promotes the process. So the tub might be the perfect strategy for helping your labor move forward.

Having said that, I don't usually encourage the tub if you're still in early labor and coping well, especially if you're hoping for a natural labor. Again, it's for mental reasons rather than physical ones. The tub is just as nice in early labor as in later labor, but it won't have the same effect on you. Let me explain why.

Jumping in the tub right away can lead you to believe that you're in the throes of active labor when you still have a ways to go. I don't want you to start the process overly excited about the small stuff. If you get too excited too early, you'll be less prepared mentally for the more challenging phases of labor when they come. If I can help you stay nonchalant and distract you from contractions in the early phases we're a long way toward helping you accomplish a natural birth. And, if you want a natural labor we have to use our best tricks strategically!

This is one reason why I hope that if you really want natural labor you won't get admitted too early. I'd love for you to get in the tub the minute you come through the door, but if you're only 2 centimeters on arrival with hours of labor ahead of you, you might get tired of the tub before things really start to percolate.

There's also a bit of a limit to the amount of time that you should spend in the tub. If you like your tub water on the hot side, spending too much time in the tub could raise your body temperature. And raising your body temperature could raise the baby's temperature and heart rate. There's also evidence that being in the tub too long could work against your body's ability to produce contractions by decreasing the level of oxytocin in your blood$_{10}$.

The tub really is a fabulous strategy for helping you cope with labor. Many women feel that contractions are much more tolerable with gallons of warm water swirling around their body. For moms who are shy about the tub I'll often negotiate by saying "How about trying it for 2 contractions and see what you think. If you don't like it you can get out." Quite often after 2 contractions they're believers! For shy moms I cover their topside with a towel or have them wear light clothing. So if this is you, remember to pack something to wear in the tub. Don't miss out on the joy of this wonderful and helpful experience.

You also have options while you're in the tub. Some women like the jets on, others like the jets off. Some like the lights on, some like them out. Some women kneel in the tub and let the shower splash warm water on their backside. Some soak submerged to their chin. Make it work for you.

Drop your shoulders

If there's one thing I see more than any other when women are in labor, it's the shoulders in the ears thing. When women hurt they hunch up their shoulders, and from there their entire body becomes rigid. This will work against you. (I'm beginning to sound like a broken record I know!) Relaxing is easier said than done, but everything we do to help women in labor is designed to promote it. Thus I'm always watching for creeping shoulders and try to coach them *down*.

The best way to do this is with that good breathing. When you blow out, let your shoulders drop. Let them sag as the contraction slides away. Picture everything rolling and moving down. Don't be afraid to make some noise when you blow out. It may not seem very ladylike, but no one cares at this point.

Touch and pressure points

Touch is not something that everyone is comfortable with, but for most women it's a wonderful strategy for helping cope with the discomforts of labor. Many women have back pain in labor and there are several reasons for this. Often it's just because you're working hard, you're nine months pregnant, and your back aches. The other common reason is related to the position of the baby's head against your tailbone. Pinpoint low back pain may indicate that the baby is facing up (occiput posterior) with the back of his or her head pushing against your tailbone.

There are several strategies for helping alleviate this. One is to have someone (the person with the strongest hands) take the heel of their hand and put it right on the spot that hurts and push. Have someone do this for you during the contraction. Steady, hard pressure (not rubbing). Let them know if you need more pressure or less. Quite often you'll want more!

Ideally we'd like to try to help the baby turn into a better position. We'll talk more about this in Chapter Five.

The other thing that can help with low back pain is to labor in forward-leaning positions: kneeling on the bed or leaning over the birthing ball. Another advantage to forward-leaning positions is that it gives your caretakers good access to your back. It's much easier to push on that sore spot if we can reach it.

It also makes it easier for someone to roll your hips. This is a little hard to describe on paper, but it's another nice strategy for helping relieve back pain. I've seen it done several ways, but the easiest way to do it is to have someone place their hands on your hips, fingers on your hip bones, thumbs pointing toward your spine and roll your hips backwards. (Picturing this I realize will take a good imagination!)

Give it a try. Like I tell everyone, if you don't like it we can do something different.

Massage is also wonderful during labor, but a word to the wise. Many women get to the point where they don't want to be touched anymore, and it's usually when you think they need it most! As things progress and become more intense, the desire for touch comes to a screeching halt. If you're worried about your normally sweet-natured bride casting unprintables your way, watch for the cues. Touching her when she's reached that "don't touch me" point can elicit some choice words. If you can't resist the urge to touch her, do so during the rest periods.

Create atmosphere

All women know how wonderful atmosphere is! Creating atmosphere is a woman's forte, so feel free to do so for your labor. Make the room a happy, soothing place. Turn the lights down low or play your favorite music in the background. Here are some other ideas:

- Bring your favorite soft blanket
- Bring your favorite slippers
- Try some nice smelling scents like lavender or citrus.
- How about putting flameless candles around the room?
- Bring pictures of your favorite people
- Drape a beautiful piece of fabric over something in the room
  (I'm a fabric-aholic, so this is my favorite!)

Have fun being creative!

Last, but not least, have someone with you who will push you through

Every woman needs a supportive person with them during labor, but if you're hoping for a natural childbirth, it's a must. That person could be your husband, sister, friend, or doula. (I'm not implying that your husband *isn't* the most supportive person, but some husbands feel a bit overwhelmed when the textbook becomes reality).

Talk with your husband about this one. My deepest hope is that your *nurse* will be your best support person, but it's possible, depending upon how she feels about natural labor, that she won't push you through the hard parts.

It'll be helpful if your chosen support person knows something about childbirth if you want a successful natural birth. I say this from experience. Even if your husband has the heart to help you, it can be hard for him to know what's normal and what's not in terms of your response to what's happening. He may feel so overwhelmed that he'll think that every bit of your labor seems abnormal! I see this in their eyes. That *"please tell me this is normal"* look. Having someone with you who can assure you both that everything is normal is helpful. Taking a good childbirth class will also help you in this department.

Of course the opposite is also true. If things *aren't* "normal," your support person needs the knowledge and expertise to guide the process into safe territory. This is why a good labor nurse is your best support person! (I confess I'm biased.)

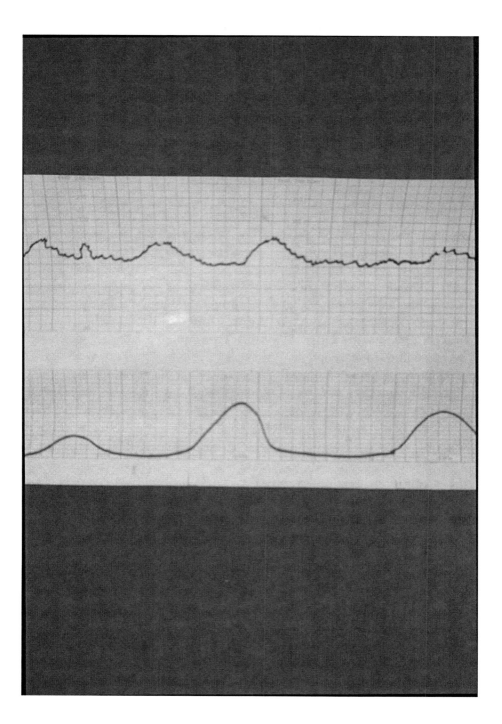

Chapter Five
The baby in labor

Normal labor is good for the normal, full-term baby. Contractions and pushing and the actual birth itself provide some very positive benefits for helping prepare your baby for life outside the uterus. The pressure that the baby takes on his or her chest during contractions and pushing helps to prepare the baby for breathing. The big squeeze that the baby gets when the head is delivered and the chest is drawn into the birth canal helps push water from the baby's lungs. All of this to help prepare baby for that first wonderful breath at delivery!

There are a lot of factors that play into how labor goes for the baby. Essentially, labor is a *stressor*, but under normal circumstances *stressor* in a *good* sort of way, like the stress athletes feel when they exercise. If you think about it, a certain degree of stress is healthy for all of us. Without some healthy stress in our lives we don't learn or grow. What we as care providers have to constantly evaluate during the process of labor is whether the stress the baby is undergoing is normal and healthy, or whether it has become *distress*. There's a big difference. And it takes experience and training to know which is which, and what to do about it.

In this chapter we're going to talk a bit about how the baby copes during labor and how we help the baby if he or she needs it. But let's start with a really fascinating topic: helping the baby get into a good position.

Positioning the baby
We spend a lot of time talking these days about why so many babies are sunny-side-up (occiput posterior or "OP"). There are a lot of theories out there on this subject, from the notion that we don't spend enough time in the garden to the belief that we spend too much time in front of the

television. It's hard to say if more babies are sunny-side-up these days than there were in the olden days since we don't have the numbers, but one thing we all agree on—a sunny-side-up baby makes for a trickier delivery.

When the baby is sunny-side-up women typically experience more back pain ("back labor"). When the baby is in a good position the contraction is usually felt low and in the front. Occiput posterior babies have a harder time engaging in the pelvis and cause the contractions to be less coordinated. This leads to longer labor and more need for oxytocin to help labor happen. Pushing an OP baby out can also be more difficult, and babies who don't turn often need help delivering with either forceps or a vacuum, or by cesarean section.

For these reasons we spend a lot of time brainstorming how we can help the OP baby turn into a better position. Before I share some ideas with you, let me say that there are a variety of factors that might impact how easily your baby can turn. Like how big he or she is or how wrapped up your baby is in the cord. You shouldn't try to force your baby to turn by pushing on your tummy. This could actually cause problems with your placenta if you happen to push on your tummy in the place where your placenta sits. The best way to help your baby turn is to try some positioning techniques and pray he or she is able to help!

It may be that your baby has been OP for weeks and won't be easily coaxed, but the time to try is before he or she drops snug into your pelvis. Of course it doesn't mean that he won't turn during labor, but helping him line up before he comes into your pelvis is a nice idea. Some suggest that just good upright posture will help him get organized. Others recommend forward-leaning positions as this will tip your pelvis forward and give your baby more room to turn.[6]

While you're still at home in the early phases of labor try kneeling in front of your sofa resting your elbows on the seat cushion. Placing a pillow under your knees will make it more comfortable for you. This will be a good time to practice relaxing your hips. Gently sway them side to side and front to back. When you rock your hips front to back tuck your bum in and then extend it up ... tuck it in, extend it up.

Working on your flexibility may also help give your baby more room to turn. Your pelvis has a number of flexible parts and as we get older our joints become less flexible. If you're an older first-time mom this may be something you can work on, but be careful. You don't want to hurt yourself by putting too much stress or strain on creaky joints and ligaments. Whatever you do, do it gently.

Research, and plain old-fashioned common sense, tells us that being upright and moving around during labor helps the baby make those tricky turns$_9$. Once you get to the hospital it's pretty common to put you in bed to monitor the baby. But it's certainly possible to monitor the baby while you're standing, so after they've checked you out feel free to get up (unless there's a reason why you shouldn't). If your baby needs continuous monitoring, ask if they have a telemetry unit. This way your nurse can monitor your baby while you move around.

But it's also ok to rest! Don't think that you're harming the situation if you want to get a nap. Resting gives you energy for the long haul. When you nap, lie on your side with as many pillows as they'll give you! Put them between your knees, hug one like a teddy-bear, and tuck one behind your back. Try moving your top leg forward over the pillow mountain and pull your bottom leg back. It's even ok to lie partially on your stomach if you have enough pillows to support you. The only position you want to avoid is reclining on your back.

When you sit try to sit as upright as you can. Also try leaning forward over a table or against your partner. You can even do many of these positions if you have an epidural. Don't let being confined to bed hinder your creativity. Of course you won't be able to stand, but your nurse, midwife or doula can help you into some really creative positions. They'll have plenty of their own good ideas too, so don't feel that you have to memorize any of these. The bottom line is you're going to do your best.

If your baby just can't seem to turn and the angle of his head is hindering descent, your doctor or midwife may be able to help. Sometimes they can turn the baby's head with their hand during labor, and sometimes they can do so at delivery with forceps. As you can imagine, this will be a little less uncomfortable with an epidural. If your baby's head hasn't come down low enough though with pushing, your doctor won't be able to help with forceps or vacuum. We'll talk a bit more about this when we talk about the pushing stage.

A life sustaining system

Plain and simple, pregnancy is a miracle. I'm forever amazed that the human race has even survived. This is because another miracle of your body—your immune system—is on the march to protect you from foreign invaders, and the fetus is definitely a foreign invader! Your DNA is different and your blood is different, making the fetus a perfect target for granulocytes and antibodies! So how does the fetus survive and thrive? Well, it's complicated. But far beyond the mysteries of the marvelous pyramids in Egypt, pregnancy tops the list of ancient wonders of the world!

Your baby interfaces with you by an amazing system of tissue and blood vessels beginning with the placenta and travelling through the umbilical cord. Through this intricate network of veins and arteries, nutrients and oxygen flow to your baby. The efficiency of this system depends upon *flow*—healthy, unrestricted, glorious **flow**.

Labor nurses are always thinking about flow to the baby and what variables may be impacting it. You might be surprised by how many variables there are! Some variables develop during pregnancy, such as the quality and character of the umbilical cord. Others are imposed, such as smoking or taking certain drugs. Here's a list of some of the variables that may hamper flow to the baby:

Inherent Variables	Imposed Variables
• Skinny umbilical cord • Short umbilical cord • Knots in the cord • Cord around the baby's neck • Placenta positioned over the cervix • High blood pressure • Diabetes • Spontaneous separation of the placenta	• Smoking • Illegal drugs like cocaine • Laying flat on your back • Severe dehydration • Severe malnutrition • Acute low blood pressure • Overuse of oxytocin • Addominal trauma causing separation of the placenta

All flow problems need consideration. But all are managed differently depending upon when they occur and to what degree (if any) the baby is compromised. Some problems we can fix and some we can't. For example, if a serious flow problem develops in the first few months of pregnancy we probably won't be able to fix it and the baby won't survive. Sadly, this will lead to miscarriage. At the other end of the spectrum, if a serious flow problem develops midway through your labor and we can't resolve it quickly, you'll be off to the c-section room for delivery.

Every baby faces potential flow problems. It's the job of your care provider to be on the lookout for problems, either during pregnancy or during labor. Do we "watch and wait" when we see evidence of a flow problem or do we jump in and deliver? Well it depends on how bad the problem is and how easy it is to fix. If you're early in your pregnancy we sure don't want to deliver the baby if we don't have to, so the goal is to help improve flow. This could mean medication, bed rest, or even hospitalization.

If poor flow of nutrients causes your baby to stop growing, your provider may indeed recommend delivery even if your baby is premature. The reason for this is that in time the placenta that stops feeding the baby will also stop oxygenating the baby, and a baby without oxygen dies. So even though no one wants to deliver a baby prematurely, a premature baby has some chance of survival. An un-oxygenated one doesn't.

Flow during labor

Flow problems can creep up on any baby regardless of oxytocin, epidurals or other interventions. During normal contractions blood flow through the placenta completely shuts off. When the contraction eases off blood flow resumes. This is the normal operation. Can the baby survive then without oxygen for a spell? Well, actually, no. One of the beautiful things about the placenta is that it holds some oxygen in reserve so that the baby can make it through the contractions. This is another reason why those rest periods between contractions are so important. It's then that blood comes surging back through the placenta giving the baby the opportunity to re-build reserves.

One issue therefore that can cause flow problems during labor is too many contractions and not enough resting. This can happen when you're receiving oxytocin. It's the nurse's job to make sure that contractions don't average more than two minutes apart so that oxygen reserves can be replenished.

Oxygen reserves can also be depleted if labor is too long. Now a good healthy placenta can go quite a while before oxygen reserves are depleted, but a placenta damaged by high blood pressure or diabetes may not. This is why we monitor the baby. A baby with good reserve will tolerate normal labor just fine, but a baby with poor reserve won't. Every baby though has a limit.

The umbilical cord also plays a critical role in oxygenating the baby because the cord is how the oxygen gets from the placenta to the baby. Every cord is a little different. Some are thick and some are thin. Some are long and some are short. Some are wrapped around a body part and some have a knot in them. (Knots happen when the baby is *really* little and swims around and through a loop).

All of these factors can impact blood flow through the cord during contractions. Thick hearty cords cope better with the pressure of contractions than skinny or knotted cords. Sometimes cords get compressed because the amniotic fluid is low and there isn't enough to cushion them effectively. We actually see evidence of cord compression during labor all the time. It's very common and if its short lived it doesn't cause the baby much trouble.

The job of your care taker (your nurse, doctor and/or midwife) is to make sure the baby is coping with labor. For the most important thing about labor is bringing the baby out full of well-oxygenated blood!

Lizzie showed up in full-blown labor! It was her first baby and she really wanted natural childbirth, so she stayed home as long as she could. She was 4 centimeters and 100% effaced when she arrived. Twenty minutes after she hit the door her bag of water broke, and then the trouble began.

We were just getting ready to take her off the monitor and put her in the tub when the baby's heart rate tracing took a turn for the worse. Big deep drops in the heart rate occurred with each contraction. We helped Lizzie turn to her other side and gave her oxygen. We started an I.V. (intra-venous catheter) to help improve flow. Nothing we did improved the situation. The heart rate pattern became more ominous with each passing minute.

The doctor examined Lizzie and found that she was now 5cm after her bag of water broke, but the baby was nowhere close. We put Lizzie on her knees and elbows and asked her to take deep slow breaths. Nothing was helping. The baby was in trouble and needed help fast.

We had no choice but to take Lizzie to the operating room to deliver her baby.

Lizzie's darling red-headed girl was born 5 minutes after we got to the operating room by low transverse c-section. She whimpered meekly as she came into the light, Apgars of 4 and 9 (at one minute and five minutes of birth respectively.) This told us that she still had good oxygen reserve, but that it had been fading fast. We all looked up as the doctor took out the placenta and showed us 5 true knots in the baby's umbilical cord!

Lizzie was so glad she got to the hospital when she did—and so were we!

Monitoring the baby

The reason we monitor the baby is so that we can watch for flow problems. If a flow problem develops the baby's heart rate pattern tells us. We feel a *great* deal of responsibility for the baby as you labor—and we should.

There are two accepted methods for monitoring the baby during labor; listening to the heart rate for a short time with a Doppler, or tracing the baby continuously[11]. When you first get to the hospital you'll be monitored continuously so that we have a baseline picture of the baby's environment. This means that you'll have two straps placed around your tummy, each one holding a monitoring device. One will track your baby, the other will track your contractions.

One little hint about the monitors. If they're sitting on your tummy (external vs. internal monitoring), the contraction device is *not* measuring the strength of the contractions. It's only *sensing* them. Like if you push your finger on your arm you can tell if you're pushing harder or softer, but you can't measure the pressure. So don't get too excited if the contraction looks like a big one. On the other hand, don't be disappointed if it looks small. The picture is subjective. (And remember, not focusing on them at all is a good labor strategy!) We aren't really looking at the numbers anyway. We're looking at the baby to see how he or she responds when the contractions happen.

Your situation will determine whether or not your baby needs to be monitored continuously or intermittently. If you have any health issues, are on oxytocin, or have an epidural you'll need continuous monitoring. If your initial tracing checks out ok, your baby can be monitored intermittently. If at any point your care takers have concerns they'll switch you back to continuous monitoring. Remember though that being monitored continuously doesn't mean that you have to be locked in bed. Feel free to be as creative as you can be within your given situation.

How we help the baby

The whole point of monitoring is to make sure that the baby tolerates the journey of labor. Continuous monitoring has taken some criticism because of the fact that care takers all respond a little differently to what they see. We all know that the world is full of "grey" and the world of healthcare is no different. We all agree when the baby looks good, but we may not agree about things that raise our concerns.

This is why studies have found that continuous monitoring increases the possibility of cesarean delivery, because we err on the side of caution. We feel that it's better to deliver the baby when he or she still has some reserve rather than wait 'til baby's tank is on empty.

If we have concerns about the baby there are numerous things that we can do to help refill the tank before we have to do a c-section. If baby responds by looking better we keep going forward. One of the first things we do is change your position. Since many flow issues relate to pressure on the cord, changing your position often helps remedy the situation. If low blood pressure is causing the problem, we lower your head and give you more IV fluid. If you're on oxytocin we can turn it down or turn it off. Contracting less may help improve flow, but it may also slow your labor progress. It's a balancing act.

Some flow issues are mild and don't cause much problem, some get worse over time. If the baby's heart tracing changes to the point where we feel that oxygen reserves are running low your provider will want to deliver you. The method of delivery will be determined by where you're at in your labor. If you've been pushing for two hours and your baby is nice and low your doctor may be able to deliver you with a vacuum or forceps. But if vaginal delivery is a long way off and your baby is getting worse, our only choice will be a c-section if we want a healthy baby.

Lastly, there are times when the baby's heart rate drops unexpectedly to a dangerously low rate—and stays there. This represents a serious flow issue. Thankfully this isn't common and most babies respond to our efforts to help. Sometimes we know what contributed to it and sometimes we don't. When it happens we work very quickly to help the baby recover. This is because we know that we only have a short time to either help the baby recover or get the baby out before oxygen deprivation sets in. If we have to do a c-section, there's a lot to do in that short time and we use every minute as efficiently as we can.

Understanding the nuances of how the baby is coping with labor takes practice and expertise. This is why we work as a team. We help each other and discuss things with each other. And we always keep the well-being of you and your baby at the heart of our care.

It was one of those days.

I responded to a code blue in the emergency room. Typically this means the team is working to help an older person suffering from a heart attack.

Today they were working frantically on a newborn infant who wasn't breathing.

One of the nurses approached a young woman standing beside me and began asking her some questions. The woman, the mother's midwife, calmly explained that her client came to the birth center at 7am at 9 centimeters dilated. She then went on to describe subsequent events giving precise information about the fetal heart rate. On several occasions, she said, it was between 60 and 90 beats per minute. She explained that she cut an episiotomy when the heart rate was 60 and delivered the baby.

None of the information she shared particularly raised any red flags. What raised that notorious red flag in my heart was the number on the clock. It was 10 pm.

Very few infants, if any, will tolerate 15 hours of labor from 9 centimeters to delivery. The impact on the baby's head and stress on blood flow through the placenta just about guarantees oxygen deprivation and neurologic damage.

This healthy looking, 9lb boy didn't live to see his second day.

The first step in fetal monitoring is knowing the difference between what's normal and what isn't.

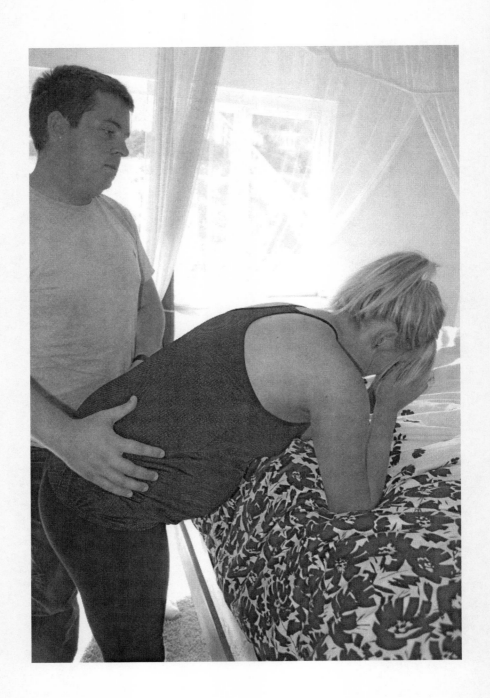

Chapter Six
Pain management options

Labor pain affects everyone a little differently. Since no one can get inside your body, who can say if the pain for you is actually different or if your ability to cope with it is just different. I think I've seen just about everything. From women who keep it all inside to those who let it all hang out. Some women don't seem to be too fazed until they're well down the road, and some struggle with the first painful contraction. In one way, though, you're all the same. You all hope for a short, minimally challenging birth. And I would love to be able to promise each one of you exactly that!

You know enough already to know that first labors are usually the longest and that there's some pain involved. This is why there are so many books and blogs that talk about creative ways for managing labor pain. I can't speak to every belief or idea out there (there are some unique ones!), so I'll just talk about a few of the most common methods used for helping women cope with the pain of labor.

Before we talk about options, let's talk a little about people and their beliefs about pain. There's a wide range of opinions out there between the pros and cons of *having* pain, and the pros and cons of *treating* pain. The beliefs people have about pain guide them in their decisions regarding how to "do" labor.

Of course, there really aren't any pros to *having* pain, but some feel that the pain of childbirth is natural and expected so they view it differently from pain generated in other ways.

You probably have strong ideas too, and if you haven't already, now's a good time to start exploring them. Many of you know already that you want an epidural—no questions asked. Some of you aren't sure what you want because you don't know what to expect and you want to keep an open mind. And some of you believe that if you don't achieve a natural, non-medicated childbirth you won't be able to look at yourself in the mirror again!

Those who care for women in labor also have feelings about pain. Like I said earlier, most of us are just hard-wired for pain relief. Seeing someone you care about in severe pain can be really tough. I think it's true, though, that midwives in general are more accepting of the pain of labor than physicians. But all of us know that pain is pain no matter where it comes from. And we believe that you have the right to have it treated if you want to. The goal in treating your pain is to maximize comfort while minimizing risks$_{12}$.

The two sides of the discussion look something like this:

- Labor pain is a normal part of childbirth
- Pain can be managed with the help of supportive people and creative strategies*
- There are risks to medical interventions such as intravenous medication and epidurals*
- Preference is to avoid additional risk
- Intravenous medication may hinder early breastfeeding attempts*
- Epidural anesthesia will increase the need for oxytocin administration*
- Epidural anesthesia may hinder early bonding*
- Epidural anesthesia prevents the opportunity to use the tub and other alternative strategies*
- Epidural anesthesia may hinder freedom of movement during the pushing stage*
- Epidural anesthesia may increase the likelihood of a forceps or vacuum delivery*

- Pain is pain no matter what causes it
- Pain can result in negative physical conditions such as hyperventilation, higher blood pressure, and over production of adrenalin in the blood stream*

- Negative physical changes can decrease blood flow to the baby*
- Women should have their pain alleviated if they choose to
- The risks of medication and epidurals are low and may outweigh the risks of pain and hysteria caused by labor and delivery*
- Epidural anesthesia can lower blood pressure caused by pain, promote relaxation and consequently improve blood flow to the baby*
- A comfortable birth may increase satisfaction and decrease the risk of post partum depression*
  (There's evidence to say that post partum depression makes it difficult for moms to bond with their babies[14].)
- Epidural anesthesia during labor may eliminate the need for general anesthesia if the need for an emergency cesarean delivery arises*

*There may be some evidence to support these statements, but each one falls within a bigger picture. For example, there's no current evidence to support the belief that epidurals in and of themselves hinder maternal-newborn bonding. An epidural may increase the risk of short-term newborn fever and a warm baby may be less interactive than a baby with a normal temperature. The relationship between epidural anesthesia and maternal-newborn interaction, therefore, may be **indirectly** related rather than directly related[13]

As you can see, this is a lively discussion with strong feelings on both sides, and both sides have their merit. Ultimately, you get to decide what experience you want to pursue, and if in the end you've accomplished the *goal* (healthy baby, healthy mommy), you've had a great experience!

Relaxation techniques

The pain you experience can be related to a number of things; how anxious you are, how the baby's positioned, how supported you feel, or how calm the people around you are. Sometimes we can help you cope better with the pain of labor even if we don't take it away. This is what relaxation techniques are designed for.

We've already talked a lot about the importance of relaxation for getting through labor and helping labor move forward. Go back and take a look at Chapter Four if you want to refresh your memory. Remember, even if you plan to have an epidural you'll experience some degree of labor before you get it. Thus, learning how to relax and work through contractions will really help you out.

Non-medicinal strategies

Doctors and nurses take a bit of criticism from birth center and home birth advocates for our apparent lack of willingness to implement alternative therapies for pain relief. I'll be the first to admit that a lot of care providers who work in-hospital are pretty attached to the epidural package. Because so many women want epidural anesthesia, there does seem to be reluctance in some quarters to try new things.

But there are other reasons why alternative therapies haven't caught on in the United States. We haven't found some of them to be overly effective and the research at this point is sketchy.

The best question to ask might be "*do these therapies help*" versus "*do they take the pain away.*" There's a difference. Most of the studies have looked at how women rate their pain instead of how women feel they benefitted. Our strategies for supporting you in labor aren't always designed to take the pain away, but to help you cope better with it. And if you're hoping for a natural labor this is an important goal. Thus, therapies like massage, acupressure, or aromatherapy might be helpful for you even if they don't eliminate the pain.

One therapy used throughout Europe and Canada is the TENS unit (the transcutaneous electrical nerve stimulator). The belief is that stimulation of the nerves in the skin of the lower back helps to alleviate the pain of labor. Studies evaluating use of the TENS unit for labor and for chronic pain either didn't show reduction in reported levels of pain or the results of the studies were unclear[8, 15]. Women who say that they would use a TENS unit again with their next labor may have benefitted psychologically from the ability to control some aspect of their experience[10].

Therapies such as acupuncture, biofeedback, hypnosis, intracutaneous sterile water injections, and respiratory autogenic training are still being studied as to their effectiveness in helping to reduce the pain of labor[16]. Reported benefits may be related to personal testimony only.

So I'll conclude this section with my own personal testimony! Women who are able to keep a strong handle on their emotions and approach labor in a meditative sort of way get through natural labor with more success.

But I certainly can't say if the meditative mind-set was the secret to their success or some other factor such as a short, straight-forward labor.

Medication

When I support women in labor I mentally strategize where we're going and how quickly we seem to be getting there. I come up with what I think will be a good plan (secretly in my mind) after having spent a while talking to my client about her hopes and dreams.

The two biggest factors I consider in determining this plan are what my client's looking for in terms of the experience, and where she's at in the process. Certain strategies are better employed early in labor and others are better employed later when things are a little tougher. The biggest challenge is trying to help those women cope who feel they're ready for the late labor strategies when they're still early in the process.

Trying to explain to my client why we should try one strategy now and wait to try another later can be tricky. But part of the explanation is that once a strategy has been tried it often doesn't work as well later. So it's best to reserve some of the better strategies for the tough times and not use them up in the early phases. This is true of pain medication.

If my client plans to have an epidural but labor hasn't really kicked in yet, I usually encourage strategies like walking, resting, rocking, and tubbing. In time, if the cervix is still only slowly changing and my client is beginning to struggle (meaning walking, rocking and tubbing have lost their appeal), it's time to talk about pain medication. Pain medication is given I.V. (intravenously) because we don't want it to stay in your system long. I.V. medication goes into your blood stream so your baby will get some of it. Most medications that we give I.V. during labor are cleared from your system within a couple of hours after administration.

Studies have shown that medication may not necessarily reduce your pain, but it can do a good job of helping you relax and get some rest between your contractions[10]. The relaxation that you get from the drug may also do wonders for helping you let your body move things forward. Once upon a time I had a client who really wanted a natural labor but got stuck at 6 centimeters. It was very discouraging for her and every other trick we tried did nothing to make her cervix budge.

Finally I suggested we try a small dose of medication. We tucked her into bed and nestled her with pillows preparing her for a nice little nap. Within 30 minutes of giving her the medication she told me she felt like pushing. She didn't get much of a nap, but just a few minutes of rest gave her the energy she needed to get through the rest of her labor without an epidural.

It won't work this way for every one of you because some of you will be truly stuck. But, for those of you who need just a bit of help relaxing your pelvis so the baby can descend, medication may be just the thing.

Every doctor has a different drug that they prefer to give. Some cause nausea and vomiting and many cause you to feel a little light headed—like you've had a tall glass of champagne! Don't fight the sedative sensation that it gives you. Relax and go with the flow. This way the medication can help you move forward better in your labor.

Because of the relaxation effect and because I.V. medication crosses over to the baby, the baby will also feel sleepy during the time the drug is in your system. When we give I.V. medication, though, we give it right in the middle of a contraction to minimize flow of the drug to the baby. The power of the contraction temporarily shuts off blood flow through the placenta, so if the drug is given during a contraction mom will get the majority of the drug and baby will get less.

If the drug you're given is a narcotic and the baby is born with some still in his or her system, the baby could need some help with breathing. This is why we try not to give you I.V. medication with an hour or so of birth. But, of course, we have no idea when birth will happen. We can only make an educated guess.

Another concern regarding I.V. medication is that we don't fully know if there are any long-term consequences for the baby. This is something that needs more study. On the positive side, the use of I.V. medication alone (and not getting an epidural) results in shorter labors, less need for oxytocin and better ability to push your baby out unassisted[10].

Two doses of medication are about the limit in terms of effectiveness. So if you're hoping to avoid an epidural but find that you need some help, strategize your doses carefully. Save them for the time when you really need them—hopefully later in labor rather than earlier!

Epidurals

What do I think about epidurals? Well, I think they're a marvelous invention of modern medicine! I think, when placed at the right time, they can do wonders for helping you feel more comfortable during your labor. One of the myths regarding epidurals though is that they take away all your pain. Truthfully, epidurals aren't designed to eliminate all of your sensation. They're designed to reduce pain so that you can rest and relax. Ideally you should still feel pressure and have an urge to push when the time comes.

Every epidural works a little differently. One friend may tell you that it worked great, and one may say that it didn't work at all. There are lots of reasons why women have different experiences. Sometimes the medication absorbs into one region more than another or sometimes labor progresses so fast after placement that the epidural has a hard time keeping up.

Epidurals are placed by anesthesiologists—doctors specializing in anesthesia. Since most women want their bottom numb for birth, the epidural is placed fairly low in your back so that the medication will spread to the nerves that cover that region. The difference between a spinal and an epidural lies in where the numbing medication is placed. Both procedures produce numbing of an area of your abdomen, bum, legs and possibly chest, depending on where in your back (north or south) the doctor injects the medication.

Picture two circles, one inside of the other. The tiny space *between* the two circles is the epidural space. Inside the *inner* circle is the spinal space. This is where the spinal fluid and spinal nerves are housed. Your spinal cord actually becomes a branchy bunch of nerves as it comes into your lower back, and it's into this area, below the actual spinal cord, that labor epidurals are placed. Thus hitting your spinal cord with a needle and causing paralysis is *extremely* unlikely.

Spinal means that the medication is placed directly into the spinal space where the spinal fluid is. *Epidural* means that the medication ends up in the epidural space—that little space just *outside* of the spinal area. So why all of this conversation about spinal and epidural? Well, for one, I think it's fascinating! And two you may end up with one or the other. Knowing what to expect will help you have realistic expectations, and realistic expectations will help you keep a happy heart.

Can you see that there'll be a big difference between the two in regards to how quickly you'll get comfortable? If the medication is placed right into the spinal space you'll feel the effects very quickly. The medication mixes with the spinal fluid and spreads to the nerves rapidly thus causing almost immediate numbing sensation. This is why the anesthesiologist will often choose spinal anesthesia for an elective c-section.

You may be asking why then don't we use spinals for labor if they work so quickly. Isn't getting pain relief *fast* the main goal? Well, getting a small dose of pain killer into the spinal space *will* make you comfortable more quickly, but the dose will wear off in about an hour or two. For most of you your labor will last longer than that. It won't be possible (or realistic) for the doctor to come and give you a spinal "shot" every two hours.

The answer to this dilemma is *epidural*. Current technology allows the doctor to place a tiny tube into the epidural space that will remain in your back the entire length of your labor. Through this tube you'll get medication on a continuous basis. Sometimes the doctor will also give you the ability to dose yourself with some medication if you feel that you need a bit more[17].

Once placed, epidurals take about 15 to 20 minutes to start working. Depending upon how "easy" your anatomy is it could take anywhere between 5 minutes and 45 minutes to place the epidural. Some backs are easy and some are hard. "Hard" backs are when the doctor has difficulty feeling the landmarks. This could be because you have a curvature in your spine from scoliosis, or because you're a bit fluffy.

One thing I do is practice with my clients what will be expected of them during placement *before* the anesthesiologist comes. This way, hopefully, we can be as helpful to him or her as possible. And being helpful is helpful! I'd have you practice the curled up position, relaxing your shoulders as you breathe slowly. I may even put my finger on the lower part of your back and have you push it away. Pushing out the lower part of your back is *really* helpful. (This is something to practice at home if **epidural** is in your plan).

In order for the anesthesiologist to place your epidural he or she needs to be able to feel the spaces between your back bones. If you have scoliosis or are full-figured, or just can't curl up effectively, it can be *very* difficult for them to feel the spaces. And at times, impossible. Placing an epidural under those circumstances could mean some guess work. So the more you can curl up and push your back out, the better.

I can't speak for all anesthesiologists, but it's possible that some of them won't be willing to try under those circumstances. It may not be prudent to start poking needles into someone's back when they have no idea where they're at with the anatomy. I've seen many anesthesiologists though make heroic effort under difficult circumstances, but sometimes they just can't do it. It's a hard situation for all of us.

There are other conditions that also make having an epidural placed a "no go." Having any sort of bleeding disorder such as low platelets will disqualify you from getting a needle in your back. Platelets enable you to form blood clots and keep you from bleeding. Conditions of pregnancy, such as ITP or HELLP syndrome cause abnormally low platelet levels and thus might make it impossible for you to receive an epidural. Does the reason make sense? If we stick a needle near your spinal column and you experience bleeding that we can't stop, you could develop a big problem in there. We won't voluntarily subject you to a problem with such potentially threatening consequences.

Do we give platelet transfusions to women with low platelets so that they can have an epidural? Not typically, because we can't predict how well your body will receive the platelet transfusion. And, over time, the platelet level will slowly drop off again. Thus, the most common way of thinking is to try other forms of pain relief rather than epidural anesthesia.

When epidurals are a good idea
There are times when an epidural is an excellent idea. If you have a heart condition or high blood pressure or any issues that might increase your risk of cesarean delivery, your doctor or midwife may well recommend one. Epidurals can help reduce strain on a weak heart and help improve blood flow through a placenta damaged by high blood pressure or preeclampsia[18].

An epidural may also be a good idea if you find yourself stuck in labor and nothing else seems to be working. Sometimes the pelvic relaxation that you get from an epidural is just what it takes to move things forward.

Placement procedure

So let's talk about how it happens. My hope is that by walking you through the fine details of the placement procedure, you'll be well prepared, and less anxious, when the time comes.

When we finally all agree that it's the right time to have your epidural placed, your nurse will begin to give you fluid into your vein. This means that before you can have your epidural, you need to have an I.V. The I.V. can be capped or "locked" until the time it's needed for fluid so that you can move around unhindered by pump and pole. But, even if you have a running I.V. you should feel free to move around as much as you like. A running I.V. should not keep you trapped in bed.

It's the nurse's job to have an idea how available the anesthesiologist is and try to have you ready about the time that he or she is ready. Typically there's only one anesthesiologist available for a certain number of patients and he or she may not be available at the exact moment that you feel that you're ready. Being ready for your epidural by having your fluid in and being positioned in bed will really help move the process along when he or she walks through your door. I assure you that when they finally get to your bedside they'll make you feel as if you are the only person in the world!

The anesthesiologist will want you positioned sitting up *really slouched*, or lying on your side *curled up tight*. Now when I say curled, I mean **curled**. Anesthesiologists all have different expectations. But, I've learned that the more I can help you wrap around your baby (whether you're sitting or side-lying), the easier it is for the doctor to find that all important space between the bones. That's why practicing ahead of time really helps.

The anesthesiologist will talk to you about the risks and benefits and make sure that having an epidural is what you really want (your obvious discomfort won't be proof enough!). He or she will want to hear you say "I do."

Since we don't put epidurals in women who are not in well-established labor (at least we shouldn't), you'll be having contractions while the epidural is being placed. I know it doesn't sound easy, but your nurse will be there to help you through. This is when good breathing is so important; breathing in a way that *relaxes your shoulders*. I can't stress this enough. Relaxing your shoulders will help you push out the lower part of

LABORING WELL

95

your back thus helping the doctor get through the bones. Getting through the bones is essential for getting the medication in!

Monitors, such as a blood pressure cuff, fetal monitor, pulse oximetry and maybe a cardiac monitor will be placed on you. The anesthesiologist will push around on your back to find the right spot. He or she will then wash your back with a cold solution, numb the skin and use the epidural needle to find the right location. You shouldn't feel much discomfort during placement, so if you do, it's ok to ask for more numbing medicine in your skin.

Once the epidural space is located, some doctors will then put a long spinal needle through the epidural needle and inject a very small amount of medication into your spinal fluid. This is called a combined spinal-epidural (CSE). Remember when we talked about the fact that medication into the spinal space works faster? Well this is one twist on the procedure that combines the benefits of both therapies. If you receive a spinal dose, you'll feel your bottom start to get warm and numb within several minutes.

Once the doctor locates the epidural space he or she then slides a *very* tiny tube into the epidural space. Numbing medication and pain killing medication are given through this catheter. The catheter remains taped to your back for the entire length of your labor.

Tubing is connected to the catheter which is then threaded through a pump that continuously gives you medication throughout the length of your labor. Many pumps also give you the ability to "self-medicate" with more medicine if you need it. The doctor programs the pump so that you get enough medication to keep you comfortable, but not enough to overdose yourself!

The dose of medication that you're given, and how well the medication absorbs, will determine how numb you get. It is true that some women feel pretty immobilized and have a hard time moving their legs after placement of an epidural. I haven't found that moms are overly bothered by this though. Most are just happy to have relief from the pain.

The full numbing effect takes about 15 to 20 minutes. You'll probably feel your toes or bottom get warm first and this is a good sign that the medication is starting to work. The medication has some tendency to spread toward gravity. For this reason, your nurse will have you turn from side to side every so often to help keep you comfortable on both sides.

We won't want you lying on your back after the epidural is placed, especially during that first hour after placement. Lying on your back compresses the large blood vessel running up your abdomen behind your baby. When this vessel is compressed it can cause a drop in your blood pressure. Epidural anesthesia may *also* cause a drop in blood pressure, and two strikes against your blood pressure won't be good for your baby. When blood pressure falls the baby gets less blood flow. When babies get less blood flow their heart rates tend to drop. We have some tricks for helping remedy this situation if it happens, but the best plan is to try to avoid it from happening at all.

Epidurals can produce a "patchy" effect meaning that some areas may feel more numb than others. If this is true for you, don't panic. It doesn't mean that your epidural isn't working. It just means that you'll need to lie on the side that's hurting to help the medication sink to that area. The ideal epidural does *not* take away all of your sensation. You should still be able to move your legs and turn yourself in bed.

From the moment that numbing medication is placed into your epidural, walking and standing will be impossible. It's important though that you continue to move into different positions while laboring with your epidural. Movement during labor is good for helping labor progress, and it's all about progress[9]! Being confined to bed will also mean that you'll either need to urinate on a bedpan or will get a bladder catheter.

Walking epidurals

You may have heard of something called a walking epidural. This term is a bit confusing in that a large number of women don't actually walk around when they have one. But the idea is that you *could* walk if you wanted to.

The concept of walking epidurals originally seemed to solve our dilemma regarding the ability to offer pain relief and keeping women mobile[19]. From personal experience though, I've found that many women want their epidural "up-graded" from the walking variety to the full-service variety fairly quickly. This is why many anesthesiologists aren't crazy about recommending them.

The primary difference between a full-service epidural and a walking epidural is the medication placed into the epidural space. Full service epidurals give you numbing medication and pain medication. If you get numbing medication you won't be able to walk. Walking epidurals give you only pain medication. (Thus the name!)

The right time

Many of us were surprised when studies came out saying that epidurals placed during early labor don't increase the risk of a c-section[20], especially when previous studies (and experience) told us otherwise. I've wrestled over whether or not to share my thoughts on this subject. For one, it's complicated and two, the issue seems settled. But, at the risk of sounding like a heretic (and because it's my book!) I'm going to offer a few thoughts on this subject.

It really goes back to our definition of labor. I've harped on this topic quite a bit already, so you all understand now that labor is not a number; it's a rate of change. In a nutshell the studies basically say that there's no greater risk for a c-section when an epidural is placed at 2 or 3cm rather than at 4cm.

The piece that's missing is whether or not we can use a number to declare that someone is in labor. We all agree that epidurals should be placed when women are "in labor." All the women in the studies may have been in labor at 2cm, but not **all** women at 2cm (or even 4cm) will be *in labor*.

If we now use a number as our guide for placing epidurals, it's quite likely we'll be placing lots of epidurals during *ripening phase*; and we do. A number doesn't distinguish between ripening phase and labor phase. And, unfortunately, there aren't studies examining the risk of c-section when epidurals are placed during ripening phase.

Factors such as how thin the cervix is, how low the baby is, and what the contractions are like are better indicators of labor than a number. I've had women in solid labor at 1cm and had no concerns about having an epidural placed. If all the factors are in "go" mode then having an epidural at any number can work to your advantage.

The simple fact is that getting an epidural *before* things are in *go-mode* just makes things harder. It's like trying to push a snowball uphill. We have to work a lot harder to get you into good labor. This means hours of oxytocin and bed rest. Since we know that movement gives the baby the best opportunity of coming straight into the pelvis[9], many are concerned about the negative implications of prolonged immobilization.

On the other hand, if the epidural is placed when the baby is low, the cervix is well effaced, and contractions are coming hard every 2-3 minutes, it's like pushing a snowball *downhill*. Things just take off! Thus I believe that you give yourself the best chance of having a vaginal birth if you use other strategies for pain management until things are in full-blown *go-forward* mode.

I watched Emma power-walk up and down the hall. Her birth plan said that she didn't want an epidural until she was at least 5cm dilated. Unfortunately, she her cervix hadn't budged past 2cm for several hours.

Her bag of water had broken 10 hours ago and her labor had been percolating for the past five. Her cervix was paper thin (100% effaced), and her baby was nearly out at a generous +2 station! Despite nice regular contractions, her cervix was just a little uncooperative.

I could see despair beginning to set in. I was trying to be support-ive of Emma's birth plan, but none of our tricks were helping move things forward. Emma was getting more tense by the minute. It was her husband who couldn't take it any longer. In private conference, they finally decided that the number didn't matter. It was time for an epidural.

Twenty minutes after her epidural was placed, Emma looked up at me with that tell-tale expression. "I think I have to push!"

Sure enough, she was 10cm dilated and her baby was +3 station! Thirty minutes later she was delivered!

She and her husband looked at each other smiling and agreed that she should have gotten her epidural two hours earlier (like I had suggested!) Even at 2cm, Emma had been in full-blown, go-forward mode.

Is it ever too late?

The answer is "yes," but every provider will have different criteria. It used to be that people said it's too late when you've reached 7 centimeters. But in truth, you could have several hours of labor ahead of you after 7 centimeters, and there's no reason to deny you pain relief during that time. Of course if you've accomplished 90% of your labor without anesthesia, you probably can do the whole thing without anesthesia! And we just might encourage you to give it a try.

In my opinion, it's too late when I think that the baby will come during the time that it takes to place the epidural (which is about 30 minutes). No one knows exactly where the finish line is so we can only make an educated guess here. But, if we know the baby is coming it's not logical to give you an epidural for the last 30 minutes of your labor.

In conclusion, *please don't lose sleep over this one.* If you're a first-time mom, it's *highly* unlikely that you'll miss your window of opportunity. The window of opportunity for first-time moms is **large!**

The culture of epidurals

Epidurals are popular, with patients and with providers. Those who are dissatisfied with the hospital model of birth feel that nurses and doctors have lost their ability to care for women wanting natural labor. They feel that we push epidural anesthesia on vulnerable and unsuspecting women.

I'll admit that hospital birth is pretty epidural-oriented. Here are some of the reasons why:

- We have excellent anesthesia services in the U.S.
- The majority of women want an epidural for labor
- Providers believe that the advantages outweigh the disadvantages
- Nurses are trained to relieve pain, thus having a patient in severe pain can be hard on them
- Epidurals allow nurses to care for more than one patient at a time if the need arises

- Epidurals give the nurse more control over the delivery, nearly guaranteeing that the doctor or midwife will be at the delivery on time
- Epidurals enable the patient to *labor-down* (see Chapter Seven)
- Many doctors believe that their ability to safely deliver the baby is enhanced when patients are calm and not moving around excessively
- Massaging the uterus after delivery to control bleeding is better performed when patients are comfortable
- Repairing any tears following delivery is easier when patients are anesthetized
- An epidural eliminates the need for general anesthesia in the event of an emergency

Some of these reasons reflect room for growth in the hospital culture. As a lover of natural childbirth, I would love to see more care providers willing and able to support women wanting natural labor. Ultimately, though, moms get to decide if they want an epidural or not. Our job is to educate them regarding their choices, and be supportive of the reasonable choices that they make.

Potential complications
Even though many women are very satisfied with their labor epidural, it's important for you to understand what issues you may face as you consider your options.

Headache
About 1% of women will get a headache following epidural anesthesia. It usually comes the day after delivery and it can be treated[17]. Sometimes it can be treated with rest and medication, and sometimes the doctor will give you a "blood patch." This means that they take a little of your blood and inject into the area of your back where the epidural was. The blood covers the leaking hole and seals it, eliminating the cause of the headache.

Infection

There's always the risk of infection when we put a needle through the skin. Epidurals are placed under sterile technique, and the doctor washes your skin with a strong cleanser to reduce the risk of infection.

Drop in blood pressure

Probably the most common problem experienced with epidural is reduced blood pressure. About 31% of women will experience a drop in blood pressure after placement of an epidural. If your blood pressure was high during pregnancy and/or labor, lower blood pressure may be a good thing for you, but your baby may react adversely to the change. Eight percent of babies will drop their heart rates in response to the reduced amount of blood flowing through the placenta[21].

This situation can often be resolved by lowering your head, giving you extra I.V. fluid, giving you oxygen or changing your position. If your baby's heart rate returns to normal quickly you can continue forward with labor. If the baby doesn't recover quickly, your doctor may perform an emergency cesarean section.

Itching

About 26% of women will experience itching with epidural anesthesia[21]. It can be treated, but even after treatment, some women still feel itchy.

Shivering (The "shakes")

Thirty one percent of women experience episodes of shivering when they have an epidural. About 10% of women shiver when they have natural labor[22]. We don't know if it's hormones, stress, or some other mechanism that causes shivering, but shivering at some point during labor is common.

Fever

About 24% of women experience fever with epidural anesthesia[21]. This risk appears to be higher for first-time moms who have long labors.

Some studies say that it's the risk of *uterine infection* that long labors present that contributes to the development of fever. Longer labors often mean your bag of water has been broken a long time, and that you've had more exams. The longer your bag is broken the greater the risk of infection and fever.

Less than 1% of babies actually have an infection even though many are evaluated[22].

Inadequate pain relief
Sometimes the epidural doesn't work the way you want it to. About 15% of women report that they weren't as comfortable as they hoped following placement of an epidural. Sometimes this can be remedied by injecting more medication or changing positions. On rare occasions the doctor will need to start again and give you a new one[21].

Longer pushing stage
Women with epidurals tend to have a longer pushing stage[23]. This may be related to the fact your urge to push is reduced. Even so, turning the epidural off for pushing isn't recommended because the nerves that control sensation come back before the nerves that control muscle strength. This means that you'll have pain before you'll have improved ability to push[19].

Increased risk for vacuum or forceps delivery
This is probably related to a longer pushing stage. The baby can only handle so much pushing, and when you reach the outer limits of acceptable pushing time frames, your doctor of midwife will recommend helping the baby out with a vacuum or forceps[23].

Increased need for oxytocin
Epidurals can slow labor down. This effect seems to be greater when placed in an earlier phase of labor rather than in

active labor. Women with epidural anesthesia often need oxytocin to help labor move forward[23].

Breastfeeding difficulties

Unlike I.V. medication, the medication given with epidurals
isn't injected into your blood stream. But it may be that a very
small amount of medication injected through the epidural gets
to the baby. Studies have found tiny amounts of medication in
newborn blood soon after birth. They've also found continuing
effects up to a couple of days after birth. This may explain why
some women feel that epidural anesthesia contributes to problems with breastfeeding, but study results are mixed[13].

Other factors may also play a part, though, in how breastfeeding goes. Babies who don't get an opportunity to start breastfeeding within the first hour of birth also seem to need more
help later. The position of your nipples (flat or pronounced) also
impacts how well babies breastfeed. Again, the effect of epidural
anesthesia on breastfeeding may be *indirect* rather than direct.
Possible long term issues need more study.

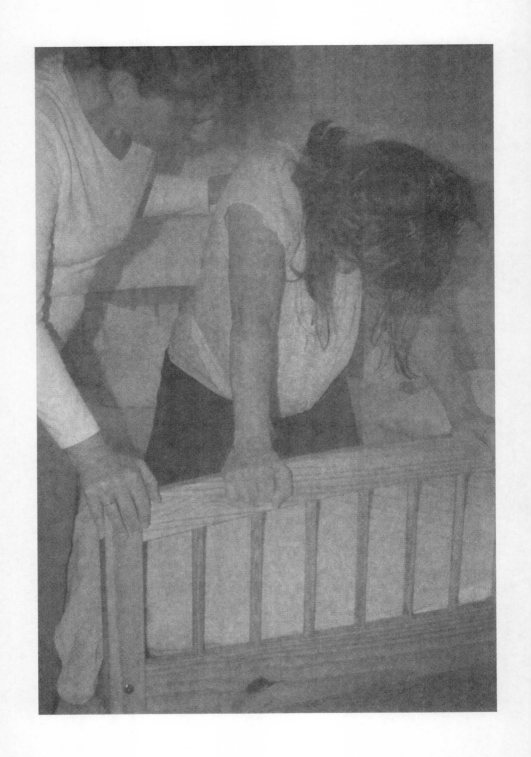

Chapter Seven
The pushing stage

In a nut shell, pushing is simply that: pushing your baby into the world. But, as you may imagine, it can take a bit of work. From your perspective, the pushing stage is really all about **GIVE**; from the baby's perspective, it's all about **FIT**. You may have heard the rumors that second, third, fourth (etc.) babies tend to come quicker—and for the most part they're true!

Once your body has been through the process before it has a better idea how to do it the next time. The reason for this is that the body is more *giving* the second or third time around. That means that things stretch more efficiently. But for *all* deliveries, the baby has to fit through the bones in order to come out. So even if you've efficiently delivered 5 babies before, fit could be a problem if number 6 is the world's next heavyweight champion!

Pushing really is more about stretch than *distance*. In reality, the baby only has a few inches to travel. If your pelvis is big enough for the baby's head, then really the work of pushing is basically about give: the more *givey* your tissues, the less work; the less *givey*, the more work.

The most challenging pushing stage I've ever experienced was with a professional ballerina. She was a beautiful girl; tall, lean … and with tissues as *givey* as concrete! Trying to push her baby's head out was like trying to push a bowling ball through pavement. The moral of the story is that you really don't need strong bottom muscles in order to have an easy birth.

Now before you start feeling anxious about the pushing stage and whether your tissues are "givey" enough, remember, if billions of women before you have done it, so can you!

The pushing stage is also called "the second stage" because, well, it comes after the first stage. (It's a very logical business.) If you remember from before, the first stage is when the cervix is dilating. Again, if you think about dilation in terms of a percentage it makes more sense. A cervix at 10 centimeters is 100% open and is no longer an obstruction in front of the baby's head. It's at this point that the pushing stage can begin.

The last little bit of cervix to disappear is often the rim just under your pubic bone. This is typically because the cervix tends to dilate where it gets most pressure (e.g. if you lay on you left side, the left side of your cervix tends to dilate more, if you lay on your right side, the right side tends to dilate more). And since women don't lie flat on their stomachs during labor (for obvious reasons!), the anterior portion tends to dilate more slowly.

Your care provider may tell you that you have an "anterior rim" or "anterior lip" ("ant lip") just before you're ready to begin your pushing stage. This just means that all of your cervix is now fully dilated *except* for that anterior portion. For some first-time moms, it could take another hour or two to get that last portion of cervix to finally disappear.

Is it necessary that all of the cervix disappear before you begin pushing?
Could a small baby come through a cervix that's only 9 centimeters dilated (or 90% open)?

Well, yes to the first, and no to the second. (Unless, you're having a very premature birth. But we're not going to talk about that scenario in this book). The answer is that for a full-term baby your cervix needs to be 100% open—or 10 centimeters dilated—before you begin pushing. Pushing against any portion of cervix can cause it to swell and that means going *backwards* in the dilation department! (Not a good thing.)

On the other hand, experienced birthers, with their lovely *givey* tissues, often possess the remarkable ability of pushing the cervix fully open from say 7 or 8 centimeters with one titanic push (sneeze, cough, puke or laugh)! If we're not on our toes, the baby comes bounding into the world before we can even get our gloves on! I have to say, though, that its times like these that make the job really fun!

Journeying through stations

Let's go back to our conversation about "stations." Like I said, the distance between them is very small. To give you some sense of how small they are, if I examine you by gently reaching in with two fingers and put them through your cervix, I can just barely feel the tippy top of your baby's head at -3 station (that's about 4 or 5 inches in). Minus 2 station is a bit lower, then -1, 0, +1, +2, and lastly +3 station as the baby moves lower in the birth canal.

The weird thing is that at +3 station the baby is not out! At +3 station we can see the top of the baby's head peeking out the vagina, but the head is far from out. To use another familiar phrase, +3 station means that you're beginning to "crown."

-3

-2

-1

-

+1

+2

+3

The only important thing to know about station is that the baby is out when it's out. That sounds extremely obvious I know, but in real life it isn't so straight forward. Pushing out your first baby can be a lot of work and many women feel that they just can't push another second. When pushing gets old, some women start asking us to help get the baby out (meaning vacuums and forceps).

I just want to give you some encouragement: you can do it! Actually, you have to. We can't just pull your baby out. And, we won't even attempt it until you've worked at it for a while and have pushed your baby down to at least +2 station. So the bulk of the work is on you. But remember, if someone can do it, you can do it! **We believe in you**.

When an inch seems like a mile

If we could create our ideal scenario with every delivery we'd love it if your baby was down to a nice low +2 or +3 station by the time we started the pushing stage. That would mean that a lot of stretching had already been done and less pushing work for you. It's very common, though, to begin your pushing stage with the head at a higher station.

Pushing stage is when we get serious about *descent*. Since the head is the biggest part of the baby, the work of pushing is getting the vagina to accommodate the head and the head to accommodate the vagina. Babies are wonderfully designed to help with *fit*. The bones of the head are soft and not fixed in place yet, so they *mold* to fit the birth canal. So don't be surprised if your baby comes out with a funny shaped head or odd looking bumps. It's all normal and in time the head will be round and beautiful again.

If your tissues are *not* givey it could take an hour or so before you begin to see some baby hair peeping out (if your baby has hair!). As the head comes lower and the tissues stretch more you'll see more and more of the top of the head. The tissues give way to the head one little step at a time until the widest part of the head is out. Once the widest part emerges, the rest of the head slips out. The shoulders are then delivered and then the rest of the baby comes out.

Some women find it really helpful to watch the pushing stage with a mirror. Seeing your baby's head so close can really motivate you! All of the work you've done to this point feels like it's really paid off. Don't be discouraged though if you watch the pushing stage and it doesn't seem like the baby is coming out. Remember it takes a while to get the tissues to give. Two steps forward, one step backward. (This is where the expression *making head-way* comes from you know!) It can take first-time moms 2 to 3 hours of pushing to give birth—with or without an epidural.

Since pushing can take its toll on both you and your baby, there are established guidelines for pushing that we consider safe. It's more likely that baby will tire of the whole business before you do, so we watch the baby closely during pushing. Our goal—our only goal—is to bring a happy, healthy baby into the world. Thus, a limit of about 3 hours of pushing is considered good practice.

If the baby isn't born after about 3 hours of pushing we begin to consider other options. If both you and your baby are still coping well, and pushing is doing the job of bringing the baby down, we'll continue to watch and wait. But, be aware of the fact that your provider is beginning to consider other options.

It's also true that if at any time during pushing (or labor) you or your baby run into serious trouble, plans will change. Remember, the important part isn't the *experience*; it's the well-being of you and your baby.

Helpful ideas for pushing

Pushing is energetic work! The vast majority of you will need to push with gusto in order to get your baby out of your womb and into your arms. And figuring out how to do it will take some practice. But no need to worry. We're here to help you and you are only going to do your best. Ideally you should begin your pushing stage when you feel the urge to push because your body then helps you know what to do. If your epidural is on the heavy side you should wait to push until you have some sense of pressure. For some women, though, that sense never comes. In this case you'll need help knowing when the contractions happen. You'll push *with* contractions and rest in between.

Helping with alignment

Just like during dilation phase, moving and changing positions is the key to helping your baby come down and out. If your baby's head still hasn't come into nice alignment with your pelvis, your care taker will suggest positions or strategies that may help. Upright positions seem to work best. If you've ever seen a picture of the old-fashioned birthing chair you can see how this "throne" position really helps point the baby's head in the right direction. Sitting on the toilet creates similar alignment. The other nice thing about sitting on the toilet or standing is that it takes pressure off your tailbone and allows your pelvis greater mobility.

If you get an epidural some upright positions won't be available to you—like standing or sitting on the toilet. But you might be able to mimic these positions by lowering the foot of the bed and raising the back. Leaning forward against the birthing ball or holding onto the squatting bar may help you keep yourself upright. Pulling on a sheet tied to the squatting bar can also help you leverage yourself while you're pushing.

Sitting straight up in bed, though, will mean that you're sitting on the "door"! It also means that your tailbone won't have as much flexibility. In order to give your baby some room and lift your bottom off the mattress try sitting on pillows. Put one length-wise under each cheek and thigh. Use as many as you need—behind your back, under your bottom ... you can't have enough pillows!

Don't be afraid to try some pushing on your knees even if you have an epidural. It takes some maneuvering, but it can really help improve pelvic flexibility. Turn yourself toward the wall, raise the back of the bed and rest yourself over some pillows. Move your hips around while you have the chance. Rock your hips back to front or sway gently side to side. Loosening things up may really help.

The important thing to remember about pushing is to try something different every so often. When women labor naturally their bodies tell them what to do. They move, they lean, they squat, they groan. *Don't be afraid to go with the flow.*

Epidurals and Laboring down

Many women with epidurals don't feel much, and that's the way they want it! Some women have a distinct urge to push with an epidural, some don't. But, even with a solid epidural you'll probably feel the pressure of the baby's head as it comes into your vagina.

What does it feel like? Well, typically it feels like you need to have a bowel movement! Lots of women wake up from a nice nap and say that they felt like they had to have a bowel movement. Instead we find that they're completely dilated and ready to push!

Laboring-down takes advantage of a nice, solid epidural. Night shift nurses invented it. If mom got her epidural at 10pm after a long day of laboring, we'd let her sleep until she felt rested, even if we knew she was 10cm dilated. We just wanted her to regain some energy before starting to push. What we found though, was that on top of having a well-rested mom, we also had a nice low baby! The pushing stage was usually shorter and easier compared to starting at *the exact* moment mom hit 10 centimeters.

Here's how you can help *laboring-down* work to your advantage. Because the baby's head coming down feels like a bowel movement, it can make women feel a little nervous. So, what they do is squeeze their bottoms with the hope of preventing stool from slipping out. But, if you squeeze your bottom, you'll also keep your baby up higher. And that defeats the whole purpose! So the secret to laboring-down is to keep your bottom relaxed and let everything slip down (and out!)

Natural pushing

Without a doubt, pushing *without* an epidural is different than pushing with one. Without an epidural your urge to push will guide the process. Many women without anesthesia feel the urge to push even *before* they're fully dilated. This is where your care taker comes in. He or she will need to let you know when it's ok to try some pushing. We really want to avoid causing the cervix to swell because that can make dilation go backwards.

If you try a push or two and the rim of cervix slides away easily, then you can begin pushing with as much gusto as you like. But if it *doesn't* and it feels tight, you'll need to try some tricks to help get you through until it slides away. Often a new position really helps. But even more important, you'll need *excellent* breathing techniques to get through this tough stage.

Try the 3 short, 1 long "pphu" that we talked about earlier. You'll really need someone to help you stay focused. You'll also need someone to help you know when the contraction finishes. Sometimes at this point you don't feel that the contraction ever finishes. But the rest period between the contractions is so important. It's at that time that both you and baby re-oxygenate. Slow your breathing *way* down and even hold it for a second or two. This will help reverse the effects of hyperventilation if you're breathing hard and fast.

Once you're given the green light to start pushing, the best thing to do is just let your body tell you what to do. Sometimes it takes a little practice—especially if you've been fighting the urge for a while. Some moms find that once they're given the green light all their desire to push fades away and they rest for a bit. That's ok. As the contractions push the baby lower, the urge to push will become undeniable.

Relaxing between contractions

Remember, you push when you're contracting and rest in between. This is how you conserve energy for the long haul. It sounds easy, but it can be tough. Switching your frame-of-mind like a light switch "on," "off," "on," "off" takes some practice. Your partner can really help you here. When you're not contracting close your eyes, take big slow breaths, let your shoulders drop *and rest*.

Resting and relaxing between contractions is also really good for the baby. Adrenalin—the hormone that gives you strength to climb mountains—also causes blood vessels to constrict. When your blood vessels constrict blood flow to the baby is reduced. Relaxing will help slow the production of adrenalin and improve blood flow to the baby. This helps keep gas in the baby's tank so that he or she has enough energy too for the long ride to the finish line.

It's also important for you to relax your legs between contractions. Women having natural childbirth will have more awareness of the aches and pains brought on by squatting or bending than a woman with an epidural. Women with epidurals need to relax their hip joints in order to prevent injury to the nerve. Have someone help you close your legs or stretch them out between contractions. This also helps shift your pelvis a bit and might help baby maneuver the corners.

Empty your Bladder

Keep your bladder empty! A full bladder can keep the baby's head from coming down, so take a trip to the toilet every now and then. If you have an epidural your care taker will help you with this if your bladder gets full.

Pushing without fear

The idea of pushing can be a little scary for women for a variety of reasons. Sometimes the first hour of pushing is only about figuring it all out and getting over your fears. One fear that plagues a lot of women is the fear of having a bowel movement while pushing. Please don't worry about this! Some of you will pass some stool, some of you won't. Your care taker will clean you up so fast you'll never know it happened!

The problem is that if you try to push in such a way as to prevent stool from coming out your baby will never come out either. You use the same muscles for pushing your baby out as you do for going to the bathroom, so you MUST push as if you're doing just that! If stool comes too, so be it. It's no big deal.

Bottom spa

On top of keeping my patients clean, I also give them the "bottom spa." When you're resting between contractions I'll take a wash cloth from a tub of warm water and gently squeeze warm water over your perineum. This can be especially comforting for women having natural childbirth. Holding the warm washcloth to your bottom can also be soothing. If your care provider hasn't tried this, ask if they would and see what you think. It may not be your thing, but it's really worth a try!

Give the baby a break

Remember, it's also important to give the baby a break while you're pushing. Resting between contractions helps re-oxygenate your baby. You might also need to breathe your way through a contraction or two if the baby is showing signs of fatigue. Women with epidurals can cease pushing with contractions much easier than women having natural childbirth.

This is why we discourage "purple pushing." Purple pushing means that you hold your breath and push hard to a slow count of 10, three times through each contraction (after which you're purple!). Over time this can lead to problems for the baby.

Now you will need to hold your breath while you push to a certain degree because that's where your power is. Think about what you do when you have a bowel movement and I think you'll see the connection. Try pushing while blowing out and see what happens. The power in your chest dissipates. If you want to get your baby *out* you need power from *within*.

The peak of the contraction only lasts for about 30 seconds and that's when you push. Push hard at the peaks and rest in between. Remember to take nice healthy, big breaths in there to keep oxygen flowing to the baby.

Preserving modesty

Those of us who experience the blessing of birth on a regular basis can forget how uncomfortable it is for some women to be seen naked. If you're someone who prefers privacy and modesty please let your care takers know. We will need to see your private areas to a certain extent during birth, but we can certainly help preserve your modesty during labor and pushing.

Is it working?

I've seen a lot of pushing in my life and the truth is some of it works and some of it doesn't. Some women get the hang of it, and others don't. Like we've discussed, it doesn't matter if every push does the job, but if over time the baby isn't coming down we'll need to try something new. It certainly helps to have a nice strong urge to push, because this helps women know how and where to focus the push.

Women without epidurals sometimes have a hard time too. This is where your care taker comes in. He or she can let you know what seems to be working and what isn't. You don't want to use up all your energy on fruitless efforts. Some women get locked into one idea because they've read or heard that it's the best strategy. But, it may be that that strategy doesn't work well for you. You can go back to that favorite strategy later because maybe it will work better after the baby has come down a bit more.

"Other options"

I hate to do it, but I need to mention just one more hard truth about labor: making it to the pushing stage doesn't guarantee a vaginal birth. I've always said that if baby's heads were shaped more like bananas than cantaloupe they'd come out a lot easier! (Maybe this is next on the evolutionary agenda.)

If three hours have come and gone and your baby still isn't born your provider will evaluate the situation. If your baby's tolerating pushing and still moving down, it'll be ok to push a little longer.

If your baby *isn't* tolerating pushing, your provider will recommend another plan. You'll be given three options. Options are dependent upon how far down your baby has come during pushing. **Unless the baby is down to at least +2 station we can't help deliver from below.** So if your baby has run out of gas and is *higher* than +2 station, the only safe option will be c-section.

If the baby is +2 station or lower the three options look like this:

1. Your provider can cut an episiotomy. Making an episiotomy gives the baby more room and may eliminate as much as an hour of pushing. When babies are in trouble, this is the quickest way to help. Depending upon how low the baby is, cutting an episiotomy may be enough to get your baby out quickly. But, some babies at +2 station won't come out with episiotomy alone, so your provider will move onto option number 2.

2. Your provider will recommend trying to deliver your baby with a vacuum device or forceps. Because of concern about the size of your baby, cutting an episiotomy typically goes hand in hand with a vacuum or forceps delivery. In all honesty, using a vacuum or forceps doesn't guarantee that we can deliver your baby vaginally. Even if your baby is +2 station, we may find that he or she is just too big to come through the birth canal.

Forceps and vacuum deliveries don't take much time because we're limited in how long we can safely try. If we've made several attempts to help the baby out, and the baby won't budge, the only option remaining is c-section. Vacuums and forceps do pose some risks. In most cases the risks are mild, like bruising on the top of the head or cheeks. Talk with your provider if you'd like more information. If you need help with a vacuum or forceps and are seeing a midwife for care, an obstetrician will be called for your delivery.

3. The last option is c-section. If the baby is +2 station and you don't want either option 1 or 2, you can say that. Since we're talking about a baby in trouble or heading for trouble here, the only remaining option then will be urgent or emergent c-section (see Chapter Nine).

The moment of birth

After 20 years of seeing babies come into the world the moment of birth still makes me emotional. There's nothing as magical as the birth of a baby.

Once your baby is born, your provider will put your baby up on your tummy. Your nurse or midwife will dry your baby off so that he or she doesn't get cold. Birth is a bit like coming out of a warm shower on a cold day. The water on their skin begins to cool them and lower their body temperature. When babies get cold they begin burning sugar to keep themselves warm, and loss of too much sugar can cause babies other problems. So, getting them dry and keeping them warm after birth is one of our priorities as we help them adjust to their new environment.

Getting your naked baby next to your warm skin is fabulous for helping him or her stay warm. And babies love it! They're often calmer next to your heart and they start thinking about eating. Ask your care takers to wait on getting your baby's weight while you and your baby get to know each other, and your baby has had time to adjust. (This might mean that you have to stifle your curiosity too!)

While you're enjoying your little one your doctor or midwife will deliver your placenta, sew up any tears and tidy you up. As soon as everything's done, you'll both be ready to give feeding a try. That first hour is the best time to give baby an opportunity. It can take some practice for both of you so don't be discouraged. Your nurse or midwife will help you. Baby isn't necessarily hungry at birth, but they're most alert. So, even if they don't have a good meal, just getting used to the nipple is a great first step.

Some babies, though, aren't quite ready for feeding right after birth because they're still trying to figure breathing out. (First things first!) Depending upon how easy or difficult your delivery was, your baby may even need some help with breathing. Sometimes the nurse can help your baby right there on your tummy. But, sometimes they need to take the baby to the warming bed in order to give the baby more help.

In time most babies get breathing figured out. But if your delivery was quite stressful for your baby, he or she may need to spend some time in the nursery getting everything figured out. It can be stressful having your baby in the nursery, but we have excellent care for babies these days. Most full-term babies are just observed for a spell and then come right back to you.

From there your adventure in parenting begins!

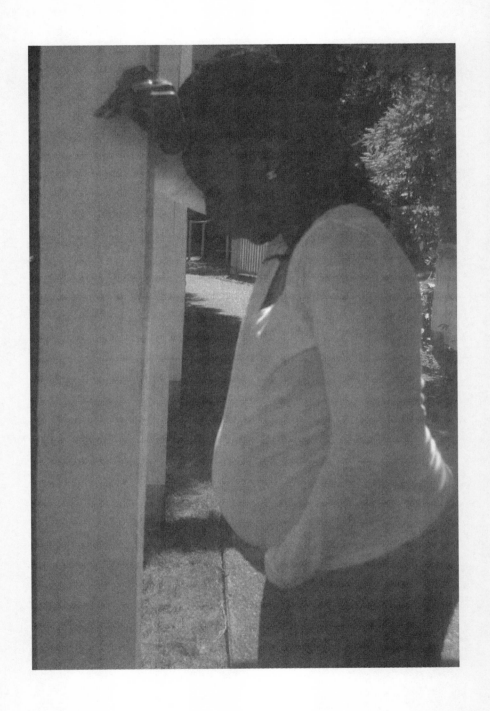

Chapter Eight
Induction of labor

Inductions of labor have been very popular. The pendulum is starting to swing back, though, because of the relationship between inducing first-time moms and the risk of c-section$_{24}$. Another problem with elective inductions has been that many babies that we *thought* were ready to come *weren't* quite ready yet. When we weigh our options on the scales, we really want to weigh them in favor of the baby. If it's better for the baby to stay in a bit longer, then that's the best option; if it's better for the baby to be born, then we pursue delivery.

One of the most common reasons that inductions occur is because moms get uncomfortable in the last few weeks of their pregnancies. It's called the T.O.B.P. induction (*"Tired Of Being Pregnant"*). If you're still early in your pregnancy as you're reading this you might think this strange. But, as your third trimester progresses, you might begin to feel a similar temptation! My well intentioned advice for you is *fight the temptation*! When it comes to labor, letting it happen when your body is ready is unarguably the best plan. So unless there's a good medical reason for induction, please don't ask for one.

The myth is that inducing labor will make the baby come out. Many moms come in very excited that *today's the day*! The problem is that we can't make the baby come out if your cervix isn't ready. It goes back to our conversation about fruit. I can't say it enough. If the fruit isn't ripe it's hard to pick! By definition induction of labor means that we'll be trying to make a process happen that hasn't decided to happen yet. And we only have so much that we can do to coax it to happen.

You know enough already to understand that you're in labor when your cervix is dilating. But, the strange truth is that we don't have any drugs to make your cervix dilate. We only have drugs to make your uterus contract. Weird, huh? The secret behind **all** labors is a cervix that can respond to the power of contractions, which is a ripe one. All too often we begin inductions when the cervix is only partially ripe, trying to squeeze a one-to-two week process into about 24 hours (or less). One way or the other, ripening needs to happen before labor can start.

Hopefully this helps you understand better why it would be best for you to wait for labor to kick in of its own free will rather than ask for an induction.

For those of you on the other side of the aisle—opposed to induction for any reason—let me say that I really appreciate how you feel. You've likely heard the rumors or are familiar with the connection between cesarean delivery and induction of labor, and you don't want one (induction or c-section!). The natural process is undoubtedly ideal, but it's also true that natural issues can creep in that make it necessary to pursue delivery to ensure the birth of a healthy baby. If this is your situation, I pray that you can feel peace about the unexpected and unwanted turn of events in your journey. This is where faith comes in—*and a clear, rational view of the goal.*

Before we talk about how we do an induction, let's chat briefly about some of the most common reasons your doctor or midwife will recommend one.

Post Dates

This means past your due date.

As you approach your due date your doctor or midwife will begin to think about a number of things, like how your cervix is ripening and how your placenta is doing. In the best of all worlds we'd love to let you stay pregnant as long as it takes to let your body do its own thing in its own sweet time. But, there are drawbacks to this idea. Sometimes there seems to be a lack of communication between the mechanisms that make labor start and your placenta. Your body may not quite be ready for labor yet, but your placenta is getting tired of doing its job!

Your placenta has a lifespan. In time it will begin to fail, shorting your baby of nutrients that he or she needs to sustain appropriate growth and well-being. If the placenta continues to fail it will also lose its ability to provide your baby with sufficient amounts of oxygen needed to support healthy brain functioning.

For these reasons, your doctor or midwife will begin to evaluate how well your placenta is functioning around the time of your due date. They may order a non-stress test (NST) or a biophysical profile ultrasound to check how the placenta is functioning. If things look good, he or she will feel all right about having you stay pregnant a while longer to see if labor kicks in on its own. They'll continue to evaluate placental functioning every few days after your due date so that they can keep a close eye on things.

Most providers will let you go about 7-10 days after your due date before they schedule you for an induction. Some are ok with two weeks, but that begins to push the outer limits of comfort. You may have heard someone say that they went 3 or even 4 weeks after their due date and didn't have any problems. My response to this is that they were either really lucky, or their dates were off.

Women are pretty good at keeping track of their periods these days, and along with early ultrasound technology we can just about pinpoint the day of conception! So, when it comes to knowing how far along you are and when you've reached the overdue point, we're usually pretty close. And it's the rare placenta that will make it to 44 weeks without putting the baby in jeopardy.

There are definite opinions out there on this topic. Some are quite critical of how conservative we've become in this department. No doubt you could find a provider who'd be more than willing to let you go longer than two weeks past your due date. My question though is *why live on the edge when it comes to the well-being of your child?*

Why would we subject babies to greater risk when we have the opportunity to avoid it? If 1 out of 1000 women lose their babies at 41 weeks and 2 out of 1000 lose them at 42_{25}, that's double the number of women who have to hear the tragic news that their baby didn't make it. And double the number of providers who have to tell them. Providers don't want to do it anymore. As you can imagine, it's the worst day of everyone's life.

Premature rupture of membranes (PROM)

Premature rupture of membranes is when your bag of water breaks before you're in labor. The word "premature" doesn't mean that your baby is premature. It just means that your bag of water broke *before* labor started. About 10% of women over 37 weeks of pregnancy will have their bag break spontaneously before labor starts[26]. Sometimes this propels you into labor, sometimes it doesn't.

Your doctor or midwife will want to check on your baby to see how he or she is coping with the change of environment when your water breaks. Someone will check your baby's heart beat and evaluate the fluid that's leaking out. (Sometimes we find that it's only urine. No need to have an emotional conversation about induction of labor if you're only leaking urine!)

If your bag is truly leaking and you're *not* having any contractions, your doctor or midwife will talk with you about a plan of action. Every provider will feel a little differently about the best way to manage premature rupture of membranes. How you all choose to proceed will depend upon a number of factors:

- Your thoughts and feelings
- How the baby is doing in the new environment
- How snug he or she is in the pelvis
- How dilated you were on your last exam
- And last, but not least, whether or not you carry *group beta strep bacteria* (GBS).

The big question will be whether to help labor get started right away, or wait to let labor kick in on its own. And if you wait, how long to wait. The risk of infection goes up with time as the warm moist (and sterile) environment of your uterus comes into contact with the warm moist (and *non-sterile*) environment of your vagina. Studies show that the risk of infection is fairly small (<10%) during the first 24 hours after your water breaks but goes up significantly after 24 hours to 40%[26].

Thus, most providers (those who appreciate the data) feel that it's a good idea to see you at least heading in the direction of labor before 24 hours.

I think some of us these days, when we hear the word *infection*, feel only mildly concerned. It may be because we've gotten so good at preventing and treating infections. We tend to take for granted the amazing progress that we've made in helping babies survive in this bug infested world. In 1900 up to 30% of infants didn't live to see their first birthday in some U.S. cities. Inability to treat infections contributed to this staggering statistic[27].

Babies are born with an immature immune system and thus are more susceptible to disease and infection. Breastfeeding certainly helps boosts baby's ability to combat certain invaders. But, if baby becomes infected while still in the uterus it won't take long, without treatment, for the baby to develop a serious and even life-threatening infection. Studies show that even when we treat the infected baby and uterus during labor the baby still has an increased risk of developing cerebral palsy[28]. All this to say that many providers would much prefer to see you delivered before you get infected. This is good care, and it makes sense.

If your cervix is nice and ripe when your water breaks you could feel labor kick in pretty quickly. But, things get a little trickier if your water breaks *before* your cervix is ripe and hasn't even started ripening yet! If you're someone who's dreaming of a certain kind of labor experience, having your bag of water break before your cervix is ripe can be a dream destroyer. It's one of those uncontrollable variables that pregnancy presents. This is when it's important to remember that the *goal* of childbirth is more important than the *experience* of childbirth. It would be wonderful if all desirable *experiences* led to the goal, but they don't.

Let's talk just a bit about how things may change for your baby when your water breaks. We like to check the baby's heart rate so we can look for signs of pressure on the umbilical cord. As water leaks out there's less cushion between the cord and other parts. Depending upon where the cord is it may get pinched as water levels decrease or when contractions occur. Even though the baby replaces some of the lost water by urinating, the rate of replacement may not be enough to provide adequate cushion. We can see evidence of this on the fetal monitor. If we see evidence of *severe* pinching we'll need to do things to help relieve the pinching, otherwise blood flow to the baby is compromised.

Sometimes the water breaks before the baby's head has come firmly into the pelvis. This leaves room for the baby's cord to slip between the head and the cervix. If this happens, it's an emergency situation called *prolapsed cord*. The baby's head can push on the cord and completely cut off blood flow. Thankfully this is a rare event, but it's another reason why your doctor or midwife will want to check things out when your water breaks.

Just two more things to mention. If you're positive for group beta strep bacteria, your provider will want to get antibiotics *and labor* going fairly quickly. Risk of the baby getting beta strep infection goes up with exposure. Since the whole process can take a while, starting everything sooner rather than later reduces baby's risk of contracting beta strep. Beta strep infection can make newborns very sick. It can cause overwhelming infection called sepsis, and/or meningitis. Both of these illnesses can cause long term disability or death$_2$.

The last thing we look for is baby bowel movement in the water (called meconium). Meconium in the water isn't always an ominous sign, but it does require some investigation$_{29}$. It could mean that the baby is feeling some degree of stress in his or her new environment or that the baby has unexpectedly shifted positions and is now coming down bottom first! Whatever the reason for the stool, we keep a close eye on these babies.

Big baby

Toward the end of your pregnancy your baby will gain about a half a pound a week. Gaining weight is a sign that your placenta is doing a good job. But, as your provider evaluates your baby's growth, he or she is also trying to consider how big of a baby you might be able to safely deliver. Baby has to fit and the tighter the fit the more risk of injury to both you and your baby.

You are all different in this department. Some of you could safely deliver an 11-pound baby, and some of you will struggle with a 6-pounder. Your provider will track how big your baby is getting by measuring your tummy or doing an ultrasound. The true test will be your journey of labor. The baby will either come out from below, or it won't. It's as simple as that.

If your provider feels that your baby is getting so big that labor and delivery may be a challenge, he or she may recommend an induction. The idea is to deliver the baby before he or she gets any bigger and help improve your chances for a vaginal birth.

Small baby

On the other end of the spectrum is the baby who stops growing. We call this baby the "growth restricted" baby. You might think it would be nice to have a small baby, but the problem with this situation is that there's usually a reason why the baby won't—or can't—grow. Sometimes we know the reason. If you have diabetes or high blood pressure, mild damage to the placenta is leading to reduced nutrition for the baby.

Sometimes, though, we don't quite know why the baby stops growing. Whatever the reason, it usually means that the placenta is failing to do its job and may be at risk for failing altogether. Babies that stop growing are at risk for a number of things including low blood sugar, low oxygen levels, and low body temperature. They also have a significantly greater risk of dying than normal full-term babies[29]. So getting these little ones delivered is a good idea.

Diabetes

Concern about *big baby* is part of the reason why your provider will recommend inducing your labor if you have diabetes. Having diabetes will mean that your baby is nourished with more sweets than the baby of non-diabetic moms, thus potentially making him or her a little chubbier. Even if your sugars have been well controlled there's the chance that your baby will be on the bigger side.

We'll talk more about diabetes in Chapter Eleven, but the primary reason for inducing diabetic moms is concern over the placenta. Diabetes damages the placenta. We've already talked about how important it is for the well-being of the baby to have a fit and healthy placenta. Because of concern over damage to the placenta and risk of early failure, doctors and midwives will very likely induce your labor before your due date if you have diabetes.

Pregnancy induced hypertension (PIH)

Some of you will develop a condition of pregnancy called pregnancy induced hypertension (again, see Chapter Eleven for more info on this topic). Pregnancy induced hypertension (PIH), and its ugly first cousins pre-eclampsia, eclampsia and HELLP syndrome, causes trouble for both mom and baby. The simple way to think about these diseases is to think of them as blood vessel wreckers. If we're able to keep your blood pressure under control we'll see less damage to blood vessels, but even so, over time it's likely that damage to small blood vessels will create problems.

Your body is full of blood vessels and all of your major organs are dependent on the nutrients and oxygen that those vessels carry. Another important organ in your body is your placenta (back to the placenta again!). When blood vessels of the placenta become damaged the baby begins to suffer.

Again, the first problem we see in this area is inadequate growth. Lack of nutrients, because of damaged blood vessels cause babies to slow or cease gaining weight. Lack of growth is a sign that baby's environment is becoming hostile. Further damage could lead to oxygen deprivation, and this could lead to neurologic damage. This is why providers recommend induction of labor for women with PIH.

Non-reassuring baby

If, for whatever reason, the baby's heart rate tracing is concerning or the baby stops moving, your provider will want to induce you. (He or she will recommend an immediate c-section if your baby is in distress!) If this is your story, expect that things will move ahead very quickly.

If a non-reassuring fetal tracing is found on a routine prenatal visit, you'll be admitted to Labor and Delivery straightaway—no going home, no passing *GO*. It's hard to understand all of the reasons why a baby may cease enjoying its cozy, hidden home. But, when we discover that this is so we know that the baby is telling us something—and we know it's time for the baby to be a newborn!

Ripening the fruit

We often get asked how long it'll take to get the baby out. And the answer is *it depends*. There are a variety of factors at play including your genes, the size of your baby, the readiness of your cervix, and the size and shape of your pelvis.

If your cervix is not quite ready or only partially ready, the first step of your induction will be to help your cervix get ready. Under natural conditions the cervix ripens very slowly, so this is where inductions can be tricky. Every cervix will respond to our efforts to promote ripening to a different degree. The degree of response is often related to how ripe the cervix was when we started. In other words a partially ripe cervix may respond nicely, while an unripe cervix may not respond at all.

Ultimately our goal is to get as much ripening as we can so that your cervix can respond to the power of contractions. The more ripening, the easier it will be to get you into labor. It's very simple (on paper that is!)

We have a number of tricks up our sleeve to help promote ripening and your doctor or midwife will have their favorite. All techniques seek to increase hormone levels either by having your body step up production, or by giving you the hormone directly in medication form.

Mechanical ripening techniques
Advantages:
- Can be done in the clinic or in Labor and Delivery.
- You might be able to go home after or with the technique
- Don't require fetal monitoring.

One easy, non-medicinal way to promote some hormone release is simply to check your cervix. Your body releases a small amount of labor hormones when we put our finger into your cervix, but it's a short lived experience.

If your cervix is open enough, your doctor or midwife might try to enhance the impact of the exam by stripping your membranes. Simply put, this means that they'll run their finger just inside your uterus and try to separate the bag of water from the wall. Needless to say this exam can be a bit uncomfortable, but on the positive side it can be quite effective in getting the show on the road$_{30}$. In spite of its effectiveness, though, sometimes it's not a good idea. Your provider may be concerned about accidentally breaking your bag of water. If you're GBS positive they won't want to risk this until you've had a dose of antibiotic on board. And you won't get antibiotics until you're admitted.

Another non-medicinal technique that's fairly popular with some providers is the balloon catheter. There's nothing special about the catheter (actually we stole it from the urology department!) But when placed into your cervix it does a pretty nice job of helping to promote ripening. Getting the catheter into your cervix can be a bit uncomfortable too, but like all our techniques, the advantages far outweigh the discomforts. (Keep telling yourself that while they're placing the catheter!)

Once the catheter is placed through your cervix the tip sits just inside your uterus. There's a balloon in the tip of the catheter that we inflate with water. The water balloon pushes down against your cervix and helps promote ripening. The catheter stays in until it falls out. This could take as long as 24hrs. I've never had anyone ask me take it out, but if you want it out, it's easy to remove. All we do is release the water and the catheter slips out.

Nipple stimulation is another technique for stimulating labor that's talked about quite a bit. This is something that women can do at home simply by rolling or placing warm clothes on their nipples. One large study found that this technique was helpful in producing contractions if the cervix was *ripe*, but wasn't helpful if the cervix wasn't ripe$_{30}$. Only low risk women were studied though, so if you have issues or complications with your pregnancy talk to your doctor or midwife before trying nipple stimulation.

Medicinal ripening techniques:
Advantages:
   • Highly effective

- Special considerations:
- Require fetal monitoring in Labor and Delivery

Medicinal techniques are all pretty similar. They all involve placing small amounts of labor promoting hormone up near your cervix. The hormone comes in the form of a gel or tablet. Once the hormone is placed, you may need to lay flat for an hour or two to give the hormone a chance to absorb. If for some reason you need to get up early to go to the bathroom you might feel the gel or tablet slide out. So be sure to go before you get your medicine!

We hope that one dose of hormone will be enough to do the job, but there are lots of times when more doses are necessary. Your doctor or midwife will explain how doses are scheduled. Doses are scheduled based on your situation. Some women will get a second dose 6 hours after the first one, and some will get a second dose the next day. If you get a second dose only 6 hours later, expect to stay in Labor and Delivery. If your provider wants to give you a second dose the next day, you may be able to go home for the night and sleep in your own bed.

Because we're artificially feeding small amounts of hormone into your system we'll need to monitor your baby for a spell. We want to make sure that your uterus (and consequently your baby) agrees with the medication. After the absorption period you'll be able to get up and move around. Once in a rare while, one dose of ripening medication will put you into labor, (sing hallelujah!) but don't expect it. Be prepared for the long haul and don't feel disappointed if it's all taking longer than you wanted. Long is normal, so don't be discouraged.

How inductions happen

Once we're ready to get contractions going, you'll officially be admitted to Labor and Delivery. You'll be placed on the fetal monitor; one monitor piece tracking contractions and one tracking the baby (or babies). Your nurse will start an I.V. and connect you to a bag of fluid. Then he or she will attach a second piece of tubing hooked to a smaller bag with oxytocin in it. Oxytocin has a powerful effect on your uterus so precise doses are monitored with a pump. This is why oxytocin is given I.V. and not some other way, because we need to have perfect control over it. That means **on** when we want it on, and **off** when we want it off.

We start oxytocin at the lowest dose and increase the dose about every 30 to 60 minutes. Depending upon how ripe and responsive your cervix is we may not need to increase it more than one or two steps. What we'll be looking for is a nice, regular, two-to-three minute contraction pattern.

Usually once we start oxytocin you'll be on it for the rest of your labor. Some people feel that once labor kicks in your body will take over and you won't need oxytocin anymore. Truthfully I haven't seen this happen very often. One possible reason for this is that if you get an epidural some of those hard earned contractions will space out. In order to keep you moving forward you'll likely need a certain amount of oxytocin. We may be able to turn it down, but turning it off completely would likely make the contractions space out and stall forward progress.

There's interesting conversation on the internet about the fact that your body feeds oxytocin into your system in a pulsatile manner and inductions feed oxytocin into your system in a continuous manner. One article states that continuously feeding oxytocin into your body doesn't give your body a break and risks jeopardizing your placenta[32]. But, this isn't true. Your body makes nice regular contractions with continuous oxytocin just as it does when labor happens naturally. We *could* make your uterus contract non-stop and jeopardize your placenta if we aren't careful, but nurses are trained to be careful and to give oxytocin appropriately.

There are a few hospitals around the country that are trialing giving oxytocin in a pulsatile manner in a way similar to the way your body gives oxytocin. It seems that this method is better at stimulating normal labor and uses less oxytocin. But, this method hasn't been found to be more effective in accomplishing vaginal birth and may lead to a longer labor[30].

Being on oxytocin doesn't mean that you have to be confined to bed. Actually moving around as naturally as possible while you're being induced is so good for you (if your condition allows it). Like we've already talked about, moving around promotes the process. It helps keep your joints limber and helps the baby maneuver the corners.

In many hospitals you can also use the bathtub when you're on oxytocin. You'll need to be connected to a telemetry monitor so that your nurse can watch your baby, but don't let this stop you. We really try to mimic a natural labor when we give oxytocin, so please don't think you have to do anything differently. Do everything you hoped to do as if you were having your own natural experience.

Your uterus is very sensitive to oxytocin so it's pretty easy to get contractions started. But you won't necessarily be uncomfortable right away. Here's an interesting fact: I can make your uterus contract—nice, beautiful, two-minute contractions—and you may not feel anything more than mild cramping. This isn't what you've heard I know. Friends have told you that an oxytocin labor is so much harder than a natural labor and here I am telling you that you may not feel anything!

Well, I didn't say that feeling nothing was a good thing! If you're not feeling anything it's probably because your cervix isn't responding to contractions yet. **Remember, we can make your uterus contract, but we can't make your cervix respond**. Depending upon the amount of ripening you got, your cervix will either respond fairly quickly to the contractions, or it won't. If it responds right away you'll start to feel discomfort right away. If it doesn't, you won't.

Thus the degree of discomfort that you feel (in a natural labor or an induced labor) is related to how well your cervix is responding to contractions. If your cervix is responding a little, you'll feel a little discomfort. If it's roaring along, you'll likely be quite uncomfortable! (The moral of the story is, if you want to be in labor, pray for pain!)

When we give oxytocin our goal is to imitate a natural contraction pattern. Our goal is to stimulate contractions that come about every two-to-three minutes. With or without oxytocin this is a normal labor pattern. Some women will dilate with contractions that come further apart, but it's rare. Since we have the technology to measure contractions, we know that contractions that cause labor to happen are the *same* strength and the *same* length as contractions that happen naturally.

During most inductions though we don't use the device that measures contractions exactly; we use external monitors on your tummy and feel the strength with our hands. The real test though of whether contractions are doing the job is progress from below. Your cervix is changing and your baby is coming down. [The device that measures the exact strength and length of contractions is called an intrauterine pressure catheter (IUPC). In order to place this catheter your cervix has to be somewhat dilated and your bag of water needs to be broken. Every situation is different in terms of the need for this sort of monitoring. The device that sits on top of your tummy isn't measuring contractions—it's *sensing* them. The contraction humps may look the same, but there's a difference in what the monitor is telling us. One tells us when contractions are happening in time, and the other tells us when they're happening in time *and* the exact pressure.]

Risks and side effects of oxytocin

As with most things in life, there are advantages and disadvantages to oxytocin. The question we have to ask is *do the advantages outweigh the disadvantages?* Because of the disadvantages, inductions should be done only because *we have to*, not because we want to. The reasons for giving oxytocin, though, extend beyond the need for inducing labor and some of the scenarios we see are tricky. In the end, the decision to give oxytocin is based upon the uniqueness of each situation.

Hopefully you've been able to see the advantages of oxytocin. Our ability to safely induce labor has improved outcomes for moms and babies. The disadvantages of oxytocin include the fact that oxytocin can make you puffy because it increases your body's ability to store fluid. High doses can lower the level of salt in your blood making your head and stomach hurt and increases your risk for nausea and vomiting.

The biggest risk of oxytocin is too many contractions. Your nurse is responsible for making sure that your uterus contracts appropriately so that oxygen reserves are not depleted[30]. What we see over time, if this happens, is changes in the baby's heart rate tracing. Often lowering the dose of oxytocin will help improve the situation. Contractions generated naturally (without oxytocin) can have the same effect on the baby. Contractions disrupt blood flow through the placenta, and *all* contractions over time—whether generated naturally or generated by oxytocin—can hinder oxygen flow to the baby. This is why there's a limit to how much labor any baby can tolerate.

The last risk I want to mention is rare, but significant. There's a very small increase in risk of the uterus tearing while getting oxytocin, but this risk is mainly in women with a scar on their uterus from prior surgery (i.e. c-section, myomectomy, etc.)[30].

Breaking your bag of water

It's quite common for your provider to break your bag of water when you're induced. Of course, like with many things, there's strong opinion about this out there on the internet. But research shows that induction is more effective by breaking your bag of water and using oxytocin at the same time[31].

Breaking your bag of water is pretty easy. The more your cervix is dilated, the easier it is for you and for your provider! Breaking your bag of water is just like an exam with the addition of another step. Once your doctor or midwife finds your cervix he or she will then reach through and scratch your bag with a sterile device, either a small plastic hook or a special glove.

When the bag has a hole in it you'll feel warm water trickling (or gushing!) from your vagina. Water will keep leaking out for the rest of your labor. Usually your provider will want to monitor the baby for a while after breaking your bag. But, having your bag broken should not limit your ability to move around, walk or use the tub. If your hope is to have a natural labor, please don't feel that anything is different. Your care takers will let you know if there's some reason why you shouldn't be mobile, but otherwise, walk around, straddle the ball, soak in the tub … and enjoy your journey!

Failed induction

Most inductions lead to vaginal birth, but for a variety of reasons they sometimes fail. We know that inducing first-time moms leads to cesarean delivery more often than spontaneous labor does[30]. This could be related to the reason for the induction in the first place—like a really big baby, or problems with the placenta. Placental problems make it harder for the baby to cope with labor. Failed induction, though, often goes back to that infamous unripe cervix. And first-time moms are most susceptible. So once again, if you're a first-time mom and are tired of being pregnant, fight the urge to ask for an induction!

If we can't get your cervix to dilate, you'll be given one of two options. We can either turn the oxytocin off and let you go home, or do a c-section.

Depending upon where you're at in your labor and the reason for the induction, going home may not be an option. If you get part-way through labor or get an epidural then c-section will be the only option. (This really won't be called a failed induction. It'll be called a c-section for *failure to progress*. We'll talk more about this in Chapter Nine.) If you spent all day contracting, but never achieved any change in your cervix, you may be given the option of going home and trying again the next day.

Of course the third option that we all discuss is *waiting longer*. We know that the first stage of labor for first-time moms is longer with an induction than with spontaneous labor$_{30}$, but care providers are all a little different in their expectations. Usually, if you demonstrate any degree of progress your doctor or midwife will let you keep working at it. How long they let you keep working at it before deciding that vaginal birth seems unlikely is a tough decision. There are a number of factors at play, and most of them are related to what's happening below. How the baby is coping with the process is also a big factor.

If your baby is still sky high after hours of labor we get a little discouraged. But this business always surprises me, and once in a while the most unlikely situation turns itself around. The cervix dilates and the baby finds the door! Only time can tell. Even so, there's a limit. If signs develop that you or your baby aren't coping with the process, the decision to deliver by c-section will be the only option for accomplishing the goal.

Miscellaneous thoughts on induction
Internet conversations

There's a lot of information on the internet about labor, birth and every other topic. It's wonderful to have so much information at our fingertips, but be careful. Some articles make interesting points, but the references used to support those points don't relate to the claims. Everyone (including me) has a particular bias. I've found that some people use arguments to promote their position without worthy evidence. For some, their own experience is evidence enough. If something worked for them it should work for everyone. But this isn't how life is. We should share our stories, but we need to be careful how our stories make others feel. Stories that subtly boast that *my way was the best way* can set others up for false expectations and painful disappointment.

If you're hoping for a natural labor and are now facing the need for induction you're probably feeling disappointed. This isn't the experience you've been dreaming of and you've heard the rumors that oxytocin makes labor harder. I hope I can encourage you. I would never tell my client who wants a natural labor that oxytocin makes labor harder, because, for one, I'm not convinced that it does!

To begin with, you can't repeat the same delivery. That "harder" labor may have been caused by something else, like a baby with a bigger head or a baby coming down with a hand by their face.

Another reason women feel that oxytocin made labor harder rests in the difference between induction of labor and *augmentation* of labor. We also give oxytocin to women who are having contractions but aren't dilating. This is called *augmentation of labor*. Here's the difference between induction of labor and augmentation of labor:

| Induction of labor | When we use oxytocin to **start** contractions |
| Augmentation of labor | When we use oxytocin to **strengthen** contractions |

Sometimes women are admitted to Labor and Delivery before their cervix is dilating. They're having painful contractions, but the contractions aren't making the cervix dilate yet. It's a dilemma for all of us. We know that they're usually still in ripening phase, but because they're tired and discouraged we offer them oxytocin to help get the show on the road. Some people may not think we should offer this option. But unless you see the tears it's hard to understand how challenging ripening phase can be for some women.

Once we start oxytocin and make the contractions more effective, the pain gets worse. This is because labor contractions hurt more than ripening contractions. The woman who gives her ripening contractions a "10" will give her labor contractions a "15." So it isn't the oxytocin per se that makes the contractions worse. It's the fact that the cervix is now responding. Once the cervix starts responding, with or without oxytocin, contractions hurt more. This is how oxytocin gets its bad name. Truly, our goal with oxytocin is to mimic a natural contraction pattern.

Self induced labor

There are lots of ideas out there about how you can get labor going. Some women have strong opinions about one idea or another (usually the one that worked for them). I have to say again that just because something worked for someone else doesn't mean it'll be the best thing for you. Women need to be careful about sharing their ideas. Some of you will feel bad if the highly acclaimed strategy doesn't work for you. Rather than saying "*Well, that just didn't work for me,*" some women ask, "*What's wrong with me?*" It's a formula for discouragement. And a heart full of discouragement is not the way to come into your labor. So be careful how you embrace all the information you hear.

There are a numerous homeopathic ideas for getting labor going, from castor oil to evening primrose. Most of the evidence supporting them is based on personal experience and personal experiences are very individual. In the final analysis *time* is the best strategy for getting labor going. Labor can even start while you're sleeping. So my best recommendation is *relax, rest,* and *be patient*. And do the things that make you happy!

The love hormone

Oxytocin is now fondly being called the "love hormone" because of what we're learning about its possible role in the initiation of maternal behaviors[33]. This latest conversation isn't doing much for calming fears or promoting happiness. Many women are now concerned that getting oxytocin may hinder their ability to bond with their baby.

Rather than getting into the nitty-gritty of the all the claims (many of which need more research) let's focus on the bigger picture.

I appreciate the belief that we use too much oxytocin, and I can appreciate efforts to steer women away from elective induction. But promoting the belief that oxytocin hinders a woman's ability to bond with her baby probably isn't the best strategy for promoting change. For one, we really don't know that it's true, and two, *is it fair?*

Women can be very sensitive. And pregnant women can be *extremely* sensitive. Any information that makes them feel that they're not doing the right thing for their baby can make them feel terrible. Most women in general are sensitive to emotional appeal, whether from stories about abused animals or ads about homeless children. This is how advertisers make their money—because emotional appeal works!

The problem with emotional appeal is that it obscures the full story. It lumps everyone and everything into the same messy dilemma. It doesn't take into account how different each situation is. When it comes to childbirth *each one is different.* From reading the blogs, you get the idea that many women think that every woman can have the same perfect experience. I wish with all my heart that it was true. But every birth is different; even the births of the same woman. The first two might be straight forward, and the third might be tricky.

We need to be very careful when it comes to using emotional appeal with expecting mothers. Some women will have no choice when it comes to inducing labor if they want a healthy baby. Many women develop problems in their pregnancy. And because our pregnant population is getting older (increasing pregnancy risks[34]) more women will face the need for induction to safeguard their baby. It isn't fair that women are being made to feel guilty by being told that oxytocin might make it difficult for them to bond with their babies.

The truth is, there are many factors that play into how well a mom bonds with her child. Mothers will bond with their babies because they *want* to bond with their babies. If you're the kind of person people like being around, it's highly likely your child will like being around you too! Happy, healthy individuals spring from happy, healthy relationships. The day that you give birth is only *one day*; your relationship with your child is for a lifetime. This should be the focus. Rather than worrying about oxytocin, study to be an excellent parent.

The love that most mothers have for their babies starts strong and then grows. It's part of who we are as women—oxytocin or no oxytocin.

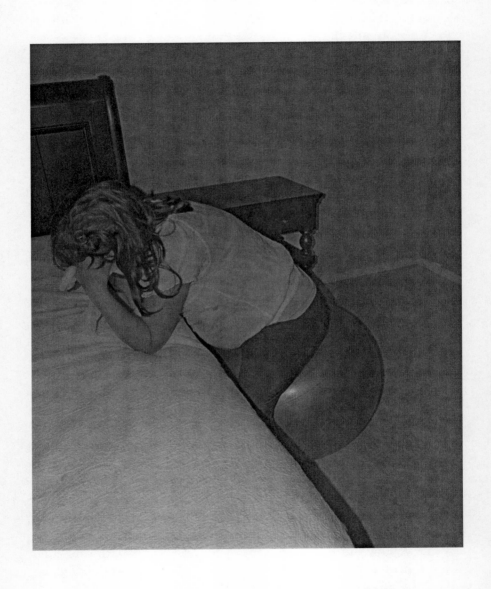

Chapter Nine
Cesarean birth

C-section rates have a lot of people in a tizzy. Without a doubt some of the rates are startling. Can't women have vaginal births anymore? Is there some evil plan afoot to pad the pockets of physicians? Certainly cesarean birth is safer than it used to be with the availability of modern anesthesia and antibiotics, but why has it become so popular? Concern over c-section is one of the reasons why some women are looking to deliver outside of the hospital.

I ask a lot of questions. In all honesty, the seemingly endless rise in rates is disturbing. One day while wrestling with this topic I asked one of my favorite obstetricians how she felt about it. I wanted to know if she thought that vaginal birth and cesarean birth were equitable deliveries. It was a provocative question (or so I thought), but one with an obvious answer.

To my surprise, though, she thought and pondered and rubbed her cheek, and ultimately said "Well, yes, yes, I think they are." (This from a woman who loves natural childbirth!)

Swallowing my dismay, I then asked, "So then you'd be ok if our c-section rate was 60%?"

"Oh no, I wouldn't be ok with that," she replied.

My dismay now graduated to full-blown confusion. There seemed to be an intellectual disconnect here! Before I could press her, though, for more of her thoughts she was called away to a delivery.

After brooding over her words for a while, a faint light began to dawn. It wasn't that she didn't feel concern over the rising rate. It was that years of experience had taught her that birth was unpredictable. And that a good c-section is better than a bad vaginal birth.

This isn't intended to worry you, but those of us who care for laboring moms and babies understand that birth is a serious matter. Most births go very well, but there's a place for c-section, even if we're all in a twitter about why the rate keeps going up. Truthfully, c-section is good news for modern woman! Talking about cesarean section is only talking about our modern and marvelous ability to deliver the baby safely should circumstances go awry.

Before we talk more about what a cesarean section is and how it happens, let's talk a bit more about factors that might be contributing to the rising rate.

Why so many c-sections?

Many people, in and out of the hospital, feel great concern over the fact that more and more women are being delivered by c-section. Haven't women been delivering babies for thousands of years? Isn't a woman's body designed for vaginal birth? Can't women take charge of their birth and safely bring forth their baby as God intended? The conversations out there on this topic are prolific and my answer is: *it's complicated.*

Let's talk for just a minute about how rates are calculated. Some people want to look at other countries or other states and make judgmental comparisons. But we have to be careful with numbers. Raw numbers don't always tell the whole story.

Take for example the place where I worked in the Middle East. We only had a cesarean section rate of 9%. We can't compare this to the U.S. rate, though, because of the extreme difference in number of babies per woman in each country. The U.S. average now is about 1.6 babies per woman. The average number of babies per woman where I worked in the Middle East was about 9. Since first-time moms have a statistically higher risk of c-section, a large percentage of women with multiple children dilutes the rate.

It's like trying to explain the divorce rate. If you have 14 married couples in the room and within the group there have been seven divorces, what's the divorce rate? I'll bet you're tempted to say the rate is 50%—and it is 50%! But now let's make Elizabeth Taylor one of the people in the room (she holds title to all 7 divorces). Do you see the rate a bit differently now? The moral is, *be careful with numbers.*

Though many of us are concerned about the rising c-section rate, we can't say what the perfect rate should be. It's wrong to try and pigeonhole society like that. It would be like trying to ask *what the perfect welfare rate should be.* We'd all like it to be zero, but we all know that in this imperfect world it isn't going to happen. We're thankful that there's a net of safety out there for those who need it.

It seems to have started in 1996. Following that year the c-section rate began to go up and up and hasn't looked back since. Is that when elective inductions became vogue? Or was there some major lawsuit that spread fear throughout the medical world? Even if we don't know for sure what pushed the rate skyward, we do know a number of things that help explain it. One of the simplest explanations is that we don't tolerate risk like we used to. We don't push moms and babies as close to the edge any-more—and that's a good thing!

What about that *get rich quick* explanation? Do doctors really do more c-sections in order to pad their pockets? In all honesty, I'm not sure I can believe that. Maybe I'm naïve. Maybe some doctors have gotten accustomed to the bigger check that cesarean delivery brings. But when you work in the trenches you see a genuine and sincere belief that surgical delivery is the right decision for the situation. The problem with the "get rich quick" view is that *nurses* often advocate for cesarean delivery even before doctors do—and nurses don't make a nickel more for cesarean birth than vaginal birth.

Without a doubt hospitals need to look more deeply into the issues and factors that are pushing c-section rates higher. And we as caretakers need to explore how we might be contributing to the rising numbers—for there's no doubt that we have a part in it all. I think there are times we could be more patient. There are times we could be less anxious. I think we could be more supportive of the natural process and recognize that not all labors are going to progress at the same rate. While I believe that these are all worthy goals, I also know that there's more to it than meets the eye. Childbirth in the modern age is a complex phenomenon.

It's not that I believe that a skillfully performed cesarean is any less of a birth experience; it's what I know about women. Most women want a vaginal birth, and cesarean delivery frightens them. Many women grieve over the loss of their dream for the sort of delivery experience that they hoped for. Thus, this is becoming a patient satisfaction issue, and lack of satisfaction is pushing women away from hospital doors.

Things have changed a lot in the world of childbirth over the years including attitudes, practices and, maybe most surprisingly, the women we serve. Many of the changes have been for the better. For example, we now believe that it's best for your baby to stay in the room with you instead of being shipped off to a nursery with large windows. We also don't make you share your room with 3 other moms like we did 20 years ago. When it comes to c-section rates, societal changes have had an impact, whether we like it or not.

Let's start with a subtle one. Overall, women don't want as many babies as they used to. Families consisting of 8, 10, 12 (or more) children weren't uncommon 100 years ago. Now that most of us live in cities we don't need as many children. Children work for you when you live on a farm, so the more the better; you work for them when you live in the city—thus two's enough!

The fact that fewer women want large families leads to *less* concern amongst physicians regarding c-section. For the woman who wants a large family, cesarean birth can be a dream-breaker. This is because a repeatedly scarred uterus faces more issues. But since women want smaller families these days, doctors feel less concerned about delivering by c-section. Doctors will opt for the choice that offers the least amount of apparent risk. While surgery certainly imposes risks, the myth is that vaginal birth does not. Vaginal birth can certainly impose significant risk to mother and baby.

A less subtle change has come in the form of litigation. More lawsuits have led to more cautious physicians and nurses, and this has impacted the c-section rate. Being cautious might be hard to understand if you've never had a job where you felt the constant threat of court. We've become a litigious society. It's part of our evolution whether we like it or not. Yet in spite of the pressure, we try to go about our jobs with smiles on our faces because we love what we do.

Have women changed?

Why is it seemingly harder and harder for women to deliver their babies vaginally? Have women really changed? If you think about it, our whole society has changed! We've experienced more change in the last 100 years than we've experienced in the previous 2000. And, yes, women have changed too.

Besides the fact that women have fewer babies, they're also waiting longer to begin having them. It's also well documented that older first-time moms have a harder time delivering vaginally than younger first-time moms. If you look at the graphs, cesarean section rates steadily rise as women get older[36]. The truth is that our most fertile years are somewhere between 20 and 30, and our best years for delivering are somewhere in there too. After that things get a bit harder. It may be true that women can have a baby later in life (with expensive, high tech medical help), but it's also true that they'll face more risks.

Another way that women have changed is that they're *bigger*. I don't mean to offend anyone, but I don't think it's a secret. We're significantly bigger. Obstetricians used to be very concerned about how much weight a woman gained during pregnancy. And women worked very hard to keep their weight gain near 20 pounds. Doctors today know what doctors knew years ago: that obesity and troubles delivering vaginally go hand-in-hand[35]. Since obstetricians are less concerned about delivering by cesarean section, maybe this explains why there's less pressure put on women to control their weight during pregnancy.

So now we have older, heavier, first-time moms. Can you see now how the c-section rate in some regards is a reflection of societal evolution?

The bigger picture

If you're someone who's appalled by the current c-section rate, it'll be hard for you to comprehend that some believe (in all sincerity) that higher cesarean rates reflect *improved* care. This is because of what they know about the alternatives! If you're someone who's had a challenging vaginal birth, you know what I mean. It would be great if every birth could be easy and perfect, but what part of life is like that? Take a look at some numbers from other parts of the globe:

Country 2010 World Health Organization data	Lifetime risk of maternal death: 1 out of every ___ women [37]	Percent of babies born by c-section. (National average [38])
Chad	15	0.4%
Ethiopia	67	1%
Pakistan	110	7%
India	170	8.5%
Ecuador	350	30%
Phillipines	300	9.5%
Egypt	490	28%
Mexico	790	38%
China	1700	26%
United States	2400	30%
United Kingdom	4600	22%
Canada	5200	26%

Do you see a trend? Do more c-sections relate to better outcomes? Maybe. But the numbers tell other stories too—like cultural attitudes, availability of resources, and number of children per mom. One take-away truth, though, is that the c-section rate will never be under 20% again.

Sadly, there are women who feel lingering sorrow—weeks, months, or years later—over the fact that they gave birth by cesarean section. I'm not sure that anything breaks my heart more than seeing tears of regret on the face of a woman rocking a gorgeous, healthy baby in her arms. Millions of women around the globe would give anything to feel the warmth of their baby close to their heart no matter how that precious package came into the world.

Is it possible that the sorrow these women suffer would be greater if a c-section had not been performed? If you're given a gorgeous, happy, and healthy baby at the end of your journey, it was all worthwhile. It's so important to keep the bigger picture in view and be thankful for the blessings of our modern age.

Now that you have lots to chew on, let's talk about how c-sections are done. One-third of you, if the rate holds true, will have your baby delivered surgically. Hopefully having some idea what to expect will make it a better experience for you.

If you need a c-section

There are three categories of c-section: scheduled, urgent and emergent. They're each a bit like they sound. Cesarean sections are scheduled for women who delivered by c-section previously and want to deliver by c-section again. If you have a placenta previa or a breech baby you'll also be scheduled for a cesarean delivery.

Urgent c-sections happen because none of our tricks are working to get your cervix to dilate or bring your baby down. These situations can be tricky. We spend a great deal of time wondering why things got stuck. Maybe it's the size of the baby, or the way the baby is coming down. Maybe immobility contributed to the situation. If you find yourself stuck, I think it's acceptable to negotiate for more time if both you and the baby are coping well. Maybe you can negotiate to have the oxytocin turned off for an hour and restarted. Maybe turning yourself into a new position every 15 minutes for an hour will help "unstick" things. We'll talk a bit more about these situations in Chapter Eleven.

Lastly, emergency c-sections are done for emergency situations. Emergency situations occur most commonly because the baby gets in trouble and *flow* is hampered. If your baby runs into trouble and we can't make him or her better quickly by turning you or giving you oxygen, you'll be whisked to the operating room for a c-section. Things happen fast because time is of the essence! Regrettably this may mean that not all of your questions get answered in full before your baby is delivered. Thankfully, true emergency c-sections are rare. If you feel the need, talk to your provider about how it all works ahead of time.

It takes a lot of people to do a c-section. If it's decided that c-section is the best way to deliver your baby the charge nurse will begin rounding up the team. It takes a surgeon, an assistant, a scrub tech, an anesthesiologist, a circulating nurse and a baby nurse to perform a c-section. If you're counting, that's six people minimum! Including you, one support person and your baby ... it's a party! You can see now why we don't let a lot of other people come into the operating room with you.

The anesthesiologist is in charge of the operating room. He or she will let you know how many people can come with you. Don't count on more than one. (On occasion though they'll agree to two). If it's an emergency situation, *no one* will be allowed to come with you. It's not because we're trying to keep things secret, it's because it's harder to take care of you and safely deliver your baby if we keep stumbling over people.

The first task at hand, before doing the c-section, is to make sure that you're comfortable. If you already have an epidural the anesthesiologist will just give you more medicine into your epidural. If you *don't* have an epidural, the team will decide how much time they have. If the situation is *emergent*, the anesthesiologist will put you to sleep. If the situation is only urgent, the anesthesiologist will give you a spinal or an epidural. With a spinal or an epidural you'll be awake to see your baby being born.

On several occasions during my time in the Middle East we had emergency situations and no anesthesiologist! I remember the first time it happened. I was so anxious about what we were going to do. But our clever obstetrician had a plan. He put numbing medicine into the skin and kept injecting until the baby came out! It was the most amazing thing. Thankfully, though, most hospitals in the U.S. have *excellent* anesthesia service, so no worries.

Because a c-section is major surgery you'll be monitored very closely. The anesthesiologist sits above your head and makes sure you're doing all right. It's not uncommon for women to feel nauseated with anesthesia. Tell the anesthesiologist if you're feeling nauseated and he or she can give you some medicine. If you have to vomit they'll help you with that too. (I know it sounds awful, but you'll be fine. Everyone is there to help you.)

After everyone is ready and everything is organized, it only takes about 10 minutes for your baby to be born. Once your baby is born the doctor will hold him or her up for you to see. It might be a little difficult for you to hold your baby skin-to-skin the moment he or she is born because of the sterile drapes. But as soon as you feel able, let your nurse know. The baby nurse takes your baby to a warming bed right near you and then brings your baby back to you once he or she's wrapped in warm blankets. Sometimes you can maneuver your arms to hold your baby, or your partner can hold your baby close for you to see.

It takes about 15-20 minutes to deliver your placenta and stitch you back together after your baby is born. The whole procedure usually takes about 30 to 40 minutes.

Once you're in the recovery room you can snuggle with your baby. The same applies to breastfeeding. It will be difficult to get started in the operating room, but once you're in the recovery room your nurse will help you get started.

Don't worry if you're lying a bit flat for your first attempt. Sitting up too quickly after surgery can trigger that pesky nausea. But the baby won't care how you're positioned. If your baby can get a nipple in his or her mouth then all is well. When moms are tired or just don't feel up to it, I help get the baby on the nipple and then let someone else take over. Your husband or a friend would be a good candidate. If your breasts are large, you'll need someone to watch the baby if you're feeling sleepy. Newborns don't have the ability to lift their heads or turn easily, so someone will need to make sure the baby is breathing while they're eating.

Most women stay in the hospital two or three nights following c-section. Since women only get one night following vaginal birth, this is one of the advantages! If gives you that much longer to recover and have people around to help you. Try to get as much rest as possible during your stay. Sleep comes in spurts when you have a new baby, so take advantage of every opportunity. And most important, enjoy your new baby!

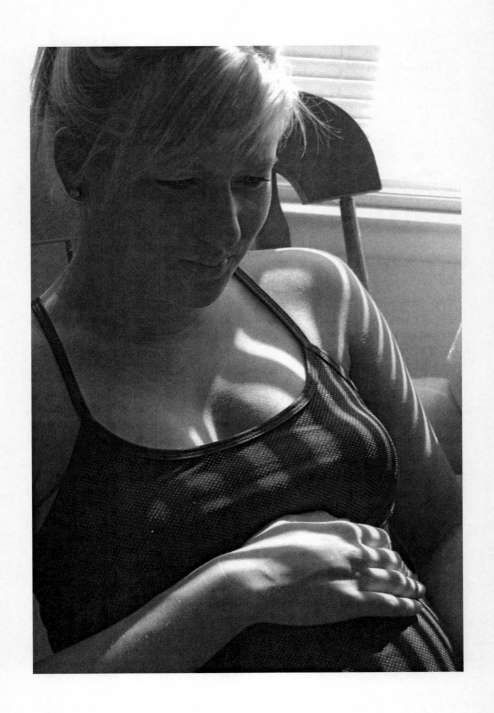

Chapter Ten
Who's who in the baby business?

There are a lot of people interested in childbirth and it can be a bit confusing sorting out who they all are. The biggest decision that you'll make for yourself and your baby will be deciding who will take care of you and where to deliver. In this chapter, I'll share a little information regarding all the different people involved in the business of childbirth. Some of these people are licensed to take care of you, and some are teachers and support people.

Doctors
Doctors are all different in their training, in their beliefs and in their experience. I've organized this chapter roughly by level of education and preparation to help you identify where people reside in the hierarchy. In the world of healthcare we always refer up the ladder if a concern or problem arises.

- *Perinatologists*

Perinatologists are doctors who specialize in high-risk obstetrics. They have the most training of anyone in the business, meaning two to three years of extra training *beyond* four years of an obstetrics residency, four years of medical school and four years of college.

They don't usually offer the same sort of service that an obstetrician or midwife does in terms of providing prenatal care and performing deliveries. Instead, they typically consult with other providers as issues arise. They offer consultation on situations such as diabetes, preeclampsia, twins or triplets, genetic diseases, and poor fetal growth. Some perinatologists even have

the ability to do surgery on the baby in the uterus! The hope is
that correcting problems before birth will improve the outcome
for the baby.

• *Obstetricians*

Obstetricians are doctors who specialize in caring for women
during pregnancy and childbirth. Their training includes four
years of college, four years of medical school and four years of
obstetrics residency before they can officially practice independently. One thing unique about obstetricians, that you may not
know, is that they're also licensed to perform surgery. Not all
doctors are licensed for surgery, and this is important when it
comes to the ability to do a cesarean section if need be.

Obstetricians also specialize in gynecology, providing care to
women throughout all realms of the female experience. Thus we
call our gynecologist an "OB/Gyn."

Obstetricians usually work together as a group because of
the nature of their job. Since they care for pregnant women,
and since babies come at any time of the day or night, obstetricians share the work of a busy practice with other obstetricians. During the day they see women in the office, and during
the night one will be "on call" to address concerns and deliver
babies.

For your prenatal care you may have one particular physician
that you see, or you may rotate through all the partners. This
gives you the opportunity to get to know them all. Even if you
see only one physician throughout your pregnancy, you may
meet the others before you deliver so that all faces are familiar.

Some women have told me that they want to see a midwife
for their pregnancy because midwives spend more time with
clients and are more in-tune with the needs of women. There
may be philosophical differences between midwives and some
obstetricians, but the time they have to give is strictly related to
how busy their practice is. If the midwife has a busy practice,
she may also have limited time to give you. Personality aside,
a better measure for choosing a good provider would be how

well they function under fire. (Thus, ask a labor nurse for a recommendation!)

In terms of being more in-tune with the needs of women, this is something that you'll have to explore on your own. People are all *so* different. In all honesty, some of the most caring, "in-tune" providers that I've worked with over the years have been *male*. This always comes as a surprise to the women I talk to. My honest opinion is, don't be afraid to consider a male obstetrician if someone recommends one.

Truthfully, what I would look for in a provider is how well they perform in the thick of a crisis. What I would want is someone who can keep their wits about them if things take a nose-dive and I or the baby need help fast. This is the most important quality in a provider.

• *Family medicine doctors*
Family medicine physicians specialize in family medicine. They offer wellness care, immunizations and disease treatment to all members of the family. These physicians complete a three year residency in family medicine following completion of medical school before taking the licensure exam. Some family medicine doctors deliver babies, some do not.

Some women like the idea of seeing a doctor for their pregnancy who can also care for them and their babies after delivery. The idea of having one doctor for the whole family is appealing. Family medicine doctors, though, will refer you to an obstetrician if concerns arise at any time during your pregnancy or labor. The obstetrician will either *consult* with your family medicine doctor, or the obstetrician will become your new doctor.

In some parts of the country family medicine doctors are the only doctors available who offer care during pregnancy and birth. Family medicine doctors in these areas have a lot of experience in the realm of birth. But in areas where obstetricians abound, family medicine doctors have less experience. Some have ceased to offer obstetric services altogether because of the inability to keep up their skills, and because of the cost of malpractice insurance.

Another thing to consider if you're going to choose a physician is the scope of their practice. Many women choose physicians because they believe that a physician can care for them in every way necessary. An important question to ask, though, is whether or not your doctor is licensed or able to perform surgery. Not all physicians are comfortable performing c-sections. So, if you're not comfortable with the idea of getting a new doctor should surgery become necessary, ask about this ahead of time.

Midwives

Sorting out midwives is a little trickier. Here in the United States there are numerous pathways for becoming a midwife, and preparation for each pathway is very different. For a nice concise overview of the differences between three of the most common pathways, search the internet for *"Comparison of Certified Nurse Midwives, Certified Midwives, and Certified Professional Midwives."* As of this writing, http://www.midwife.org/Our-Credentials offers a great chart discussing the differences between the three in terms of education, licensure, and scope of practice.

It will be really helpful to our understanding of midwives if we define two terms: certification and licensure. **Certification** is a credential added to a degree or designated training pathway that says that an individual has met certain standards, and has passed a certification exam. Midwives who graduate from a university based midwifery program are certified by the American Midwifery Certification Board (AMCB). Midwives who are trained in other ways can seek certification by showing proof of training and taking the certification exam given by the North American Registry of Midwives (NARM). University trained midwives may also be certified by NARM.

Licensure is something done by states. Licensure allows the midwife to practice midwifery in that state legally. As of this writing, only 21 states license *un-certified* midwives[39], and only 26 states license midwives certified by NARM[40]. Licensure for midwives certified by the AMCB also varies by state. This takes us into our next section. (Hold onto your hat! It is a little confusing.)

- *Certified nurse midwives and certified midwives*

In a nutshell, people entering midwifery training either have a degree in nursing or they don't have a degree in nursing.

Those who start as nurses have a Bachelors of Science degree in Nursing (BSN). At the point that they want to become midwives, they enter graduate school at a university and specialize in midwifery. Some of those nurses have worked in the realm of obstetrics prior to entering graduate school and some have worked in other clinical areas such as orthopedics or psychiatry. There are no requirements stating that one must have expertise in obstetrics before entering a graduate program in midwifery.

It's also possible to enter a graduate program in midwifery at a university with a degree in something *other* than nursing—such as biology or economics. The training, certification and licensure for these two groups is the same, but they must call themselves something different upon graduation. The nurse group calls themselves *Certified Nurse Midwives (CNM)* and the non-nurse group calls themselves *Certified Midwives (CM)*. There are substantially more Certified Nurse Midwives in the U.S. than there are Certified Midwives.

Both Certified Nurse Midwives and Certified Midwives practice on the same level as Nurse Practitioners by licensure. They have the ability to provide care during the prenatal period, perform deliveries and give on-going gynecologic care after delivery. They typically work in medical clinics and deliver babies in the hospital. Some CNM's perform deliveries in out-of-hospital settings. One thing that makes them unique is that they can write prescriptions for medications just like a Nurse Practitioner.

CNM's and CM's also typically have a pre-established relationship with an obstetrician should consultation and referral become necessary.

Both groups are certified by the AMCB following passage of the certification exam, but only Certified Nurse Midwives (CNM's) are licensed to practice midwifery in all 50 states. As of 2007, Certified Midwives (CM's) were licensed to practice only in New York, New Jersey and Rhode Island. They're authorized, but not licensed, to practice in Delaware and Missouri[41]. Prior medical education and training as a nurse contributes to states acceptance of CNM's.

- *Certified professional midwives*

A national certification credential for midwives entering practice from alternative backgrounds and educational pathways was finalized in 1994. As of 2012 NARM has now certified over 2000 midwives nationally following successful completion of a certification exam. These midwives are called Certified Professional Midwives (CPM's) and they are licensed to practice midwifery in 26 states[40].

Midwives who receive certification from NARM come from a variety of educational backgrounds. Some have studied midwifery in other countries, some have attended a formal training program and some have developed their own course of study. NARM recognizes and values a wide range of educational pathways from formal training to self study. All candidates for certification though must demonstrate entry-level competency before taking the certification exam[40].

Certified Professional Midwives are trained to deliver low-risk women in homes and birth centers. They provide care to women during the prenatal period, labor and birth, and after delivery. They also provide initial care to the newborn. CPM's typically work independently, and professional relationship with a physician willing to assume care in an emergency may or may not exist. CPM's are not licensed to write prescriptions for medication.

- *Licensed midwives*

Licensed Midwives (LM's) follow similar educational pathways (workshops, apprenticeships, formal programs) as Certified Professional Midwives. The difference between the two is that Licensed Midwives, whether by choice or lack of satisfactory qualifications, have not taken a national certification exam. Twenty one states license un-certified midwives.

Licensed Midwives predominantly deliver in homes and practice independently. In most states they are not required to have any formal relationship with a physician[39].

• *Other midwives*
At present in the United States, anyone can call themselves a midwife. There are some who offer midwifery service without a license or certification and have entered practice self-taught via books and seminars[42]. These midwives are often called "lay" midwives. They typically practice without any relationship with a physician[39].

Before moving onto nurses, I want to offer you a word of advice. Please check out any claim to relationship with a physician very carefully. Does the physician see the relationship in the way that the midwife describes it? Is the physician an obstetrician? Does he or she have admitting privileges at the nearest hospital? Will he or she accept liability for your care should transfer become necessary? It may be that your midwife sent you to a physician for an ultrasound or consultation. But, this doesn't mean that that physician can or will take care of you at the hospital should an emergency arise.

Ease and efficiency of transfer of care will be greatly impacted by the nature of the relationship between the physician and the midwife. It's a myth to believe that the nearest obstetrician will accept you under any circumstances. We'll talk more about this in Chapter Twelve.

Nurses

Nurses also fall into a variety of categories. Some are clinical specialists whose job it is to keep practices and policies current and up-to-date. Some are educators focusing on the training and development of care-giving nurses, and some are bedside nurses. Bedside nurses are the ones who actually take care of you. All practicing nurses are licensed by the state to give care.

Labor and Delivery nurses are predominantly registered nurses (RN's). This means that they have a degree in nursing from a university or

community college and have taken an exam. Specialty training for pro-
spective labor nurses happens in the classroom and at the bedside in partnership with an experienced labor nurse. Many nurses come into Labor
and Delivery having prior experience in other clinical areas such as post-
partum or emergency room. The profession of nursing also offers certification to nurses in their chosen field of specialty. Many labor nurses are
certified in labor and childbirth.

All labor nurses are trained to care for laboring women and their babies
in low-risk and high-risk situations. Most are trained to care for women
and babies in all possible scenarios as they work in tandem with a physician or CNM.

Labor nurses function in a manner similar to midwives in supporting,
coaching and evaluating women and babies during labor and the pushing phases of childbirth. Though labor nurses are authorized to perform
unexpected deliveries, they're not licensed to do so. Labor nurses work in
partnership with a physician or midwife at delivery, and assist the delivering provider in any way necessary.

Childbirth educators

Childbirth educators offer education regarding labor and birth to pro-
spective parents. There are no specific requirements necessary for becoming a childbirth educator. Some educators teach classes in private settings,
some teach in the hospital as part of the hospital community education
program. Many childbirth educators have taken a certification exam.

Training to become a childbirth educator usually involves reading
books and attending seminars. Some childbirth educators have experienced birth beyond their own, but birth experience is not required before
seeking certification. There are several organizations that certify childbirth
educators, each with their own unique philosophy and requirements.

Doulas

A doula is a woman who loves childbirth. There are no universally accepted
requirements for becoming a doula. Certification is available after gaining
some experience and taking an exam. Doulas are not required to have any

medical training and are often self-taught. The primary role of a doula is to help women feel comfortable during the journey of labor and birth. They can help with positioning and breathing and offer warm words of encouragement. Some doulas also help with breastfeeding and childcare after delivery when you go home.

Doulas primarily serve women delivering in the home or in a birth center, but are able to come to the hospital too. They are hired and paid for privately. Some insurance companies can be billed for their service. Doulas have no medical or legal responsibility for the well-being of you or your baby during the process of birth. Their role is strictly supportive[43].

Some final thoughts about doulas

I want to share just a little more information about doulas since their role is fairly recent.

As the culture of childbirth evolved, and nurses were given more responsibility, the role of doula emerged. Some women came to believe that nurses were too busy to stay with them throughout their labor, and that they were less likely to support their hopes for an un-medicated birth. Women began to hire doulas because they wanted someone to be with them and encourage their pursuit of a natural labor.

Research also found that women who had a supportive person with them continuously experienced more positive results. Women had shorter labors, needed less oxytocin and were more likely to have a spontaneous vaginal birth[44]. Rather than believing that the nurse could be this supportive person, some felt that a new role was needed. Women wanted someone specifically dedicated to the roles of coaching and comforting.

I have to give you a peek into my heart at this point. I shouldn't take it personally, but the belief that labor nurses can't fulfill the roles of coaching and comforting while also giving *care* makes me sad. Many of us have dedicated our lives to this very thing, and we've dedicated our lives to doing it well.

I've worked with some wonderful doulas, but when my patient comes in with one, my role often changes. The message I get is that I won't be the designated coach, and patients often defer to their doula for the information and help that they need. I understand how this happens, but the situation can become precarious if the two of us don't see eye-to-eye.

Many doulas have strong opinions about hospital birth, even if they lack the education to critique. Some even come with an agenda. It may be that some hospitals have room to grow, but it won't be helpful to your experience if you have a doula with an adversarial attitude. If you choose to deliver in the hospital, the doctors and nurses who care for you are medically and legally responsible for you. And contrary to some thinking, many doctors and nurses are very supportive of natural labor and love supporting women in their pursuit.

Once upon a time I had a client with a rare condition. Her baby's umbilical cord had developed in a way that put the baby at risk for hemorrhaging. The situation didn't mean that we needed to do a cesarean section on admission, but it did mean that I needed to watch the baby carefully. Since this particular client wanted a natural labor, she had hired a doula to assist her.

The doula made it clear that she thought that my desire to continuously monitor the baby was ridiculous. I explained my rationale but it only fell on deaf ears. Subtly, she continued to challenge me each step of the way. As much as I tried to be pleasant and friendly, the atmosphere was tense.

At one point, I left the room to gather supplies. While I was gone the doula took my patient off the monitors and put her in the bathtub. She felt that we had monitored the baby enough and she wanted her client to soak unencumbered by belts and monitor pieces.

It wasn't a pretty situation. The doula was asked to leave and the patient and her husband felt awkward. I tell you this because you need to know that if your doula interferes in your care, the hospital has the right to dismiss her. No one wants this sort of situation to tarnish your happy day. So, let's hope that your doula (if you hire one) understands her proper role and functions as a positive advocate for your birth experience.

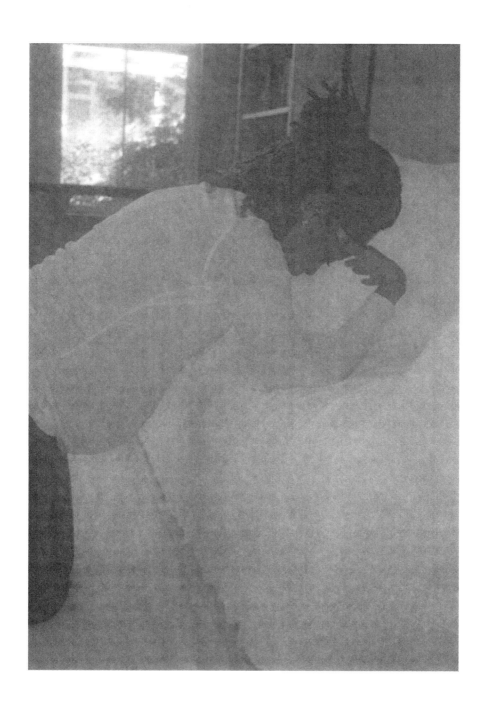

Chapter Eleven
Things that complicate labor

We all wish that things in life would always go well—especially when it comes to pregnancy. But, the fact that problems sometimes creep in explains why pregnancy, like life, is a faith experience. We're so blessed in this country to have excellent health care. We're fortunate to have providers who genuinely care for us. Prenatal care has helped improve the situation for moms and babies and has made it possible for more women to successfully deliver a healthy baby.

Things that complicate labor come in many forms. Let's start with one might not be so obvious.

- *Obesity*

    This is a very sensitive complication. We know that we're getting bigger as a society, and we know that getting bigger can predispose us to problems. But *knowing* doesn't necessarily lead to *doing*. (I speak from personal experience!)

    Obesity can impact both pregnancy and labor. Of course, pregnancy isn't the time to begin a radical diet, but pregnancy is a good time to seriously consider developing healthy, new habits. We pass our habits onto our children. So for their sakes, as well as yours, learning new ways in this area of your life could mean the difference between living well and living handicapped.

    Besides increasing the risk of daily discomforts such as back and joint pain, obesity sets pregnant women up for a number of other problems. Diabetes, high blood pressure, and blood clots are all problems that stem from obesity. Overweight women are also more likely to have large babies and difficult deliveries. Big babies are harder to deliver than normal size babies, so if your baby is big you face greater risk of cesarean delivery[45].

I realize that if you're eight months pregnant and struggle with your weight you won't be able to do much to change your situation before you deliver. But it's never too late to start taking positive steps—even if they're baby steps! Set yourself up for success and don't be discouraged. Do the things that you can stick with, even if it's one little thing. All positive steps are cause for celebration, and in time they'll become your new habits.

- **_Blood pressure disorders_**

   There's a family of problems that occur during pregnancy that cause your blood pressure to go up. Have you wondered why your doctor or midwife checks your blood pressure every time you visit? They're trending the numbers. They're watching for signs of gestational hypertension or one of other more serious blood pressure disorders.

   The problem with high blood pressure is that, over time, it can damage your blood vessels. Damaged blood vessels create problems for the tissues and organs that they serve. When blood vessels get damaged they can become leaky, scarred or form clots. With pregnancy, damage to the vessels of the placenta leads us to feel concern about how well the placenta is serving the baby.

   Another blood pressure disorder of pregnancy is called preeclampsia. Preeclampsia is when you have high blood pressure _and_ protein in your urine during the last half of your pregnancy. Normal healthy kidneys don't spill protein into the urine. Protein in your urine indicates that the blood vessels of the kidneys have become leaky due to damage. When protein shows up in your urine, your provider will know that the disease process is beginning to have a negative effect on your kidneys. They will also think that other organs may be experiencing damage too.

   Preeclampsia can progress slowly or rapidly. The earlier in pregnancy that preeclampsia develops the more rapidly it will develop and the more severe it will become. The only cure for preeclampsia is delivery of the baby. As you can see, we have many things to consider if you develop preeclampsia[46].

About 8% of women worldwide develop preeclampsia. Fifteen to 25% of women who have gestational hypertension will go on to develop preeclampsia[47]. The following groups of women have a higher risk for developing preeclampsia:

- First-time moms or moms with a new partner
- Moms who've had preeclampsia before
- Moms with a close family member with a history of preeclampsia
- Moms with twins or triplets
- Older moms
- Moms with pre-pregnancy diabetes
- Moms with pre-pregnancy high blood pressure
- Moms with a body mass index greater than 26
- And others[46]

A diagnosis of preeclampsia can make you feel emotional. No one wants to hear that a problem has developed during their pregnancy. But for the sake of yourself and your baby, a diagnosis of preeclampsia has to be taken seriously. You may not feel any different when you're first diagnosed and may feel fully capable of carrying on with your normal routine. But in time, because of the progressive nature of the disease, you might begin to feel bad.

About 25% of women diagnosed with preeclampsia will become quite sick. Preeclampsia can cause headaches, blurry vision, belly pain and nausea and vomiting. Some women experience shortness of breath, kidney failure and poor fetal growth[46]. If you notice any of these symptoms, you'll need to call your doctor or midwife right away.

During prenatal visits your provider will examine you thoroughly. They'll check your blood pressure and test your urine and reflexes. They'll weigh you to see how much water you might be retaining, draw your blood and listen to your baby. As you get closer to your due date they'll do an ultrasound to make sure your baby is growing and that everything is fine with the placenta. It's likely if you're seeing a midwife for your prenatal care he or she will refer you to a doctor for evaluation.

All the data they collect is trended to give them a picture of how the disease is advancing. If the disease is advancing slowly you'll be allowed to continue on, but probably with some restrictions. If you have a busy, stressful job, your provider will probably encourage you to stop working or slow the pace way down. This will be the time to catch up on your favorite movies, read a favorite book or take up knitting!

If the picture begins to show that the disease is progressing rapidly or you or your baby develops concerning signs, you'll be admitted to the hospital. Your provider may admit you as a short stay patient for more intensive testing, or he or she may admit you for the rest of your pregnancy.

Because of fluid retention in the brain, preeclampsia predisposes you to seizures. If you show signs that you might be at risk for a seizure, you'll be given a medication called magnesium sulfate to reduce the risk. Magnesium sulfate is only given I.V., so will require hospitalization and continuous monitoring of you and your baby. If preeclampsia worsens early in your pregnancy you'll also be given medication to help prepare your baby for birth. This is only precautionary. Your care takers will do everything they can to keep your baby in as long as possible. But if you or your baby deteriorates and you need to be delivered, you'll be prepared.

Method of delivery will be determined by a variety of factors. Labor can be induced if you and your baby can take the added stress. But if your provider thinks that you or your baby won't be able to handle the stress of labor or you need to deliver quickly, then c-section will be recommended.

Once you're delivered your body will begin to recover. The swelling will go down and your blood pressure will return to normal. If you had high blood pressure before you got pregnant, though, you'll likely need to continue medication after you deliver to keep your blood pressure at safe numbers.

Depending upon how early your baby was delivered, he or she may need to spend some time in the nursery. This won't be easy for you. It's hard to see your baby in the nursery surrounded by glass, wires and monitors. You may have to fight the urge to blame yourself for the things that your baby's going through. But, you'll have to tell yourself that you couldn't help getting preeclampsia and couldn't control how it progressed. You'll need to trust that your baby is getting the very best care known to man.

- ### *Gestational Diabetes*

One of the fascinating things about pregnancy is how your body adjusts to provide for your developing baby. You probably noticed when you got pregnant that your breasts got a little bigger. This is your body's way of getting ready to feed your baby after birth. Your body also makes changes to help feed your baby while he or she is on the *inside*. Your placenta produces hormones that raise the level of sugar in your blood making more sugar available for the baby. A little sugar for you, a little for the baby. As they say, you're eating for two!

The problem is that some women can't process the increased levels of sugar effectively and this causes high blood sugar levels (a.k.a. diabetes). It's estimated that 2% to 10% of women develop diabetes during pregnancy. If the pregnant population continues to get older and heavier it's likely that we'll see more gestational (pregnancy) diabetes[48]. Like preeclampsia, chronically high blood sugar levels can cause damage to blood vessels. We now know what that can do. For this reason, your doctor or midwife will keep a close eye on you and your baby if you have any form of diabetes.

Quite often gestational diabetes can be controlled with diet and exercise. Eating well and taking good care of yourself will benefit both you and your baby, both now and later. Gestational diabetes increases the risk that both you and your baby will get diabetes later in life[49].

Talk to your doctor or midwife about ways you can improve your diet. Remember, any positive change is cause for celebration. He or she will also have ideas for you about exercise. If you didn't exercise much before you got pregnant, pregnancy isn't the time to take up an energetic exercise program. Starting with something simple (like walking) might be helpful in bringing blood sugar levels down.

Some women with gestational diabetes have a hard time controlling blood sugar levels and need to take insulin. I know the idea of taking insulin sounds horrible, but it's better than the alternative. Diabetic women in general are at higher risk for growing really big babies. But poorly controlled diabetic women are at greater risk for other problems such as preeclampsia and stillbirth. And newborns of poorly controlled diabetic moms can struggle with issues such as respiratory distress and jaundice after they're born[49].

Deciding when and how to deliver you will involve several pieces of information. Your doctor or midwife will keep close track of how well the placenta is serving your baby and how big your baby seems to be getting. When the scales tip from *"it's better to keep the baby in"* to *"it's better to get the baby out"* your provider will discuss your options. It's very common for diabetic moms to be induced before their due date. This is because of the damage that diabetes causes the placenta and because of how big the baby gets.

Determining the baby's weight is always a bit of a guess, but we can get close. If you're 5'2" and your baby's estimated weight is 10 pounds, your provider will likely recommend cesarean delivery. Does it mean that you absolutely could not deliver a 10 pound baby? No. But learning that you can't give birth to a 10 pound baby in the midst of your delivery usually isn't a pretty site. Cesarean is recommended only when we believe that vaginal birth may present significant trauma to you and/or your baby.

Big babies predispose moms to significant tears and bleeding. Big babies are also more likely to be injured themselves. The shoulders can get stuck and this can lead to nerve damage or broken bones in the baby's shoulder. Even more significantly, if the baby's shoulders get stuck oxygen deprivation can set in if we can't deliver the baby quickly.

Once you're delivered, your blood sugars should return to normal pretty quickly. Your baby, on the other hand, may need some attention.

Babies born to diabetic mothers have to learn to control their own blood sugars after delivery. While inside you, your baby fed on a nice sugary diet. Since your insulin doesn't cross the placenta, your baby had to manufacture his or her own based upon the amount of sugar that came through. Once the free meals come to an end they'll need to slow down production of insulin. They'll also have to find a way to manufacture sugar on their own. While all of this is happening, they can run seriously low blood sugars. And seriously low blood sugars can cause babies problems.

Breathing is another problem that some baby's of diabetic moms have. This is because the increased amounts of insulin that the baby produces cause the baby to under-manufacture the substance needed for lung development. Babies who struggle with breathing after delivery will need oxygen and monitoring. It probably goes without saying that sugar and oxygen are both necessary for healthy brain functioning. But, in case this is new information for you, this is why we keep a really close eye on babies born to diabetic moms.

- *Twins*

Twin pregnancies are fascinating. And, they're on the rise! One in every 30 babies born in the United States in 2009 was a twin, compared to 1 in every 53 born in 1980—a 76% increase. One of the reasons for this is that women giving birth in 2009 were older, and older women have a higher likelihood of having twins[50]. This is because women over 35 are more likely to pass two eggs when they ovulate. Not only this, older women also get more help getting pregnant, meaning fertility medication and in-vitro fertilization. Both of these measures add to the likelihood of a twin pregnancy.

Since there are similarities between twin pregnancies and pregnancies with more babies I'm just going to talk about twins.

There are two kinds of twin pregnancies. One in which two eggs are released and fertilized (called fraternal or *non*-identical twins), and one in which just *one* egg is released and fertilized. The second case becomes twins when that one fertilized egg splits into two genetically identical embryos—thus creating identical twins.

This is where it gets interesting. Depending upon when the egg splits, one of four possible scenarios occurs. The last two scenarios are extremely rare, but if one of them becomes your situation it'll impact how we manage your pregnancy and your delivery.

A simple way to explain these four scenarios is to describe them from the perspective of the bag of water. The bag of water around your baby (or babies) has two layers, one called the chorion and one called the amnion. The timing of the split of that one egg will determine how the bags are arranged around your babies.

In the first scenario each baby has its own placenta and its own two-layer bag (this is also the situation for non-identical twins). In the second scenario there are two small bags (each housing a baby) inside one large bag. In this case the babies share one placenta. In the third scenario, both babies are in one large two-layer bag sharing one placenta. In the last scenario they share one two-layer bag, one placenta and a body part. The last scenario is called *conjoined twins*.

If your babies are together in the same two-layer bag they have some chance of getting their cords tangled as they swim around together. Because of this your doctor may want to admit you to the hospital as early as 25 weeks of pregnancy so that we can watch your babies. Now I realize that this sounds like a horrific situation—every piece of it. The idea of living at the hospital for weeks is overwhelming, let alone thinking about carrying babies at risk for tangling their umbilical cords. If this is your situation, you'll need all the family support that you can get. Your doctor doesn't mean to make your life miserable. He or she only wants the best for you and your babies.

Twin scenarios number three and number four will be delivered by cesarean section. Scenarios one and two may be delivered vaginally, but even with babies in separate bags, all twin
deliveries face unique challenges[51]. Thus no one should consider
delivering twins outside of the hospital. Women 100 years ago
may have done so, but that's because they had no other choice.
And because they didn't have a choice, they were more accepting
of life's painful consequences.

Twin pregnancies pose some unique issues. In order to see
you all through to a healthy conclusion, you'll need extra attention during your pregnancy. Twin pregnancies increase your
risk of getting preeclampsia. Some believe that preeclampsia
develops because the baby's tissue is foreign[52]. Two babies present more foreign tissue to your body, so this may explain the
increased risk. Early delivery is another risk that twin pregnancies face. We're not quite sure why this is, but one theory says
that your uterus gets stretched to the size of a nine month pregnancy *earlier*.

Your doctor will watch for signs of preterm labor and when
they do an ultrasound they'll measure the length of your cervix
to see if it's beginning to thin. If you show signs of preterm labor
your doctor will want you to slow things down. They may also
have you take medication. If preterm labor is really a threat,
your doctor will likely admit you to the hospital for bed rest
and stronger medication. You might also get a shot of medication that helps prepare your babies lungs for breathing in case
preterm labor leads to preterm birth.

Signs of preterm labor include cramping, mucusy discharge
or even some bleeding. You might feel that the babies have
dropped or have an increased sense of pressure below. But,
sometimes you won't feel that anything is different and your
doctor informs you that your cervix is thinning.

We work very hard to keep twins from delivering prematurely because premature babies are at risk for a number of
problems. They may need help with breathing, eating and staying warm depending upon how small they are at birth. Moms
often ask when they can take their babies home after they're

born prematurely. The answer is when they can manage all their important jobs, like breathing, eating and staying warm. The textbook answer though is *around your due date*. So if they come 8 weeks early, expect them to be in the nursery about 8 weeks; if they're quick learners, maybe less.

I was getting the room ready for my next patient when she walked through the door.

But the woman who walked through the door wasn't the woman I was expecting.

The first thing my new patient told me (through her tears) was that she didn't have a doctor and hadn't seen anyone during her pregnancy. One look at Shannon's face told me that her first visit with a doctor would be on the day of her delivery.

I helped Shannon undress and quickly asked her some key questions. How many babies had she delivered? Did she remember when her last period was? When did her contractions start? (etc.) As I listened to the baby's heart beat and felt her tummy I mentally calculated that she was probably about 32 or 33 weeks pregnant (7 or 8 weeks premature).

The small boy who arrived with her was her only child. He was delivered vaginally 8 years ago.

Since Shannon was a bit fluffy it was hard to feel how the baby was situated in her uterus, but it felt fairly good sized, so I was optimistic. Contractions were coming very quickly and soon after she walked through the door she started making sounds like she wanted to push! The charge nurse called the newborn intensive care team to let them know that we had an unknown baby on the way. The on-call doctor was 5 minutes out.

A gentle exam revealed that Shannon was 8cm dilated with a big, bulging bag of water. I couldn't feel a baby on the other side of the bag.

The NICU team started setting up as the doctor walked through the door. He introduced himself to Shannon, but I don't think she heard. She was oblivious to anything other than the intensity of her contractions and the pressure she was feeling below. I held her hand

and dabbed her face with a cool cloth. Despite everything, she was doing extremely well.

Dr. Kiley washed his hands and put on gloves. Just as he reached the foot of Shannon's bed, her big, bulging bag of water burst. Everything in its path became saturated with amniotic fluid— including Dr. Kiley's pants! Dr. Kiley lifted the sheet in time to see the top of a small dark-haired head coming out. He gently delivered a squirmy, noisy little boy. We all smiled in relief as he bellowed his displeasure. He looked about 32 weeks of age.

A peaceful hush filled the room as soon as the NICU team went to the nursery with Shannon's adorable little boy. Shannon lay there quietly, shocked, I think, by how quickly it all happened and by the fact that she just delivered a premature baby. I told her how beautifully she'd done. I gave her a hug, then turned to do some much needed paperwork. Dr. Kiley was waiting for the placenta.

Quietly behind me I heard Dr. Kiley say, "There's feet." I spun around to look at him. I knew he was kidding. He was known for his quiet dry sense of humor.

"You're kidding," I said.

"There's feet," he repeated as he stared at me blankly from across the bed.

I turned and ran frantically to the door hollering, "We have another baby coming!" We had nothing set up and the NICU team was busy settling baby number one.

*You've never seen people move so fast. People who work Labor and Delivery know how to do things **fast**. By the time baby number two emerged—a feisty little girl—we were ready. The shocked look on Shannon's face turned to radiant joy as she realized that she just delivered twins. Her joy was complete when she realized that she also delivered a much hoped for baby girl.*

So to summarize, there are fraternal twins, identical twins— and surprise twins!

- ***Problems with the placenta***

  Problems with the placenta come in a variety of forms. We've already talked about how the placenta can be damaged by pre-eclampsia and diabetes and how that can affect that baby's ability to cope with labor. Let's talk about a few more things that cause problems for labor and birth related to the placenta.

Placenta previa

Placenta previa is when the placenta lands over the opening of the cervix. Usually the placenta implants high in the uterus, but sometimes it implants low. I think of this as the baby that just about didn't make it! This baby was the egg that got fertilized late in its journey and just narrowly escaped being passed with the next period.

Sometimes a low lying placenta moves up and away from your cervix as your uterus grows, but sometimes it doesn't. Women with placenta previa often have issues with bleeding during pregnancy. Sometimes the bleeding is so severe that the baby is born prematurely. Women that tend to bleed often find themselves admitted to the hospital a time or two.

Bleeding during pregnancy can be horribly frightening, but in many cases the baby does just fine. If the bleeding doesn't stop with bed rest and/or medications or your baby shows signs of compromise, your doctor will deliver you.

If the placenta fully covers the cervix the only option for delivery is c-section. I think this makes sense. It's impossible for the baby to come through the cervix if the placenta blocks the way.

Placenta abruption

This is when the placenta separates from the wall of the uterus *while you're still pregnant*. There could be a number of reasons for this: trauma, cocaine use or uncontrolled high blood pressure. Sometimes we don't know why it happens. Depending upon the degree of separation the baby will either be all right or the baby will be in trouble. If the baby is in trouble, we'll need to deliver.

Sometimes you see bleeding when the placenta separates, sometimes you don't. If the placenta is high in your uterus the bleeding caused by the separation may be internal. But, most moms feel that something isn't right. They might feel mild pain or cramping, or they might feel extreme pain. Any of these symptoms should be an automatic phone call to your doctor or midwife.

Sometimes the placenta separates during labor. It's not common, but it's something that we watch for. If the abruption is serious and the baby is compromised, you'll be delivered by c-section. A woman with a mild abruption, though, can progress through to a vaginal birth and deliver a healthy, happy baby.

Retained placenta
This problem happens after the baby is delivered. It simply means that the placenta won't come out like expected. It's difficult to predict who will have a retained placenta. We know, though, that a woman with a scar on her uterus from a prior c-section will have an increased risk if the placenta happens to implant over the scar.

The vast majority of women naturally deliver their placentas within about 10 minutes after the birth of their baby. Studies have shown that the risk of post partum hemorrhage rises the longer the placenta stays in$_{53}$. The placenta can take as long as 20 to 30 minutes to come out, but after 30 minutes there's concern that the placenta is retained and that serious bleeding will result.

Bleeding with retained placenta is usually sudden and continuous. Hemorrhage after delivery is an obstetric emergency. It's been found that the average amount of blood loss with retained placenta is over 2.5 liters and this blood is lost very quickly. Over 25% of women who bleed need care in the intensive care unit[54].

Post partum hemorrhage (caused by retained pieces of placenta or ineffective contracting of the uterus following delivery) is still the number one cause of maternal death worldwide. So, providers are very concerned when the placenta is retained. There are several things we do to get the retained placenta out. One of the first things we try is to have you empty your bladder (or we'll empty it for you). Your choice will be catheter or bedpan. You won't be able to walk to the toilet if you're hemorrhaging.

Sometimes a retained placenta will come out with medication. We might give you medicine into your vein or into the umbilical vein of the retained placenta. Sometimes the doctor or midwife can remove the placenta with their hand[55]. Leaving the placenta in to reabsorb on its own is something that some people discuss, but this can only be done if there's no significant bleeding. But, bleeding with retained placenta is very common. In some cases, bleeding is so severe that the only way to stop it is to remove the uterus. This is truly a last ditch effort to save the life of the mother, and thankfully it doesn't happen very often.

You can see why it's important to have experienced staff and all the necessary equipment and medication promptly available in the event of a retained placenta.

- *Failure to progress*
  This complication happens when you stop making forward progress after you've been in the active phase of labor. There's a lot of talk about applying the same criteria to all moms in regards to rate of progression. Historically we've expected women in the active phase of labor to dilate an average of about one centimeter every hour. We're getting more flexible about this these

days, but even with less rigid expectations, the c-section rate continues to rise.

It's possible that impatience with slow labor progression contributes to this diagnosis. But how long should we wait? Sometimes I think we're very patient and sometimes I think we could have waited a little longer. When you're at the bedside, though, and your patient has been laboring in the hospital for 18, 22 or 34 hours, she's ready to be delivered.

Why women get stuck in labor is the million dollar question. Every woman and every birth is different, so it's hard to point fingers and say *"that's the reason."* There's a lot of speculation about how the institutional, packaged approach to labor may contribute to the diagnosis of failure to progress and thus to the c-section rate. Did the epidural play a part? Would more creative positioning have helped? Did we exhaust the uterus with too much oxytocin? I think these are valid questions and worthy of lively, intelligent discussion. But in the end, all anyone really wants is a happy outcome.

- ### Head-pelvic disproportion (CPD)

The diagnosis of *cephalo-pelvic disproportion* is similar to the diagnosis of failure to progress. It's just a fancy way of saying that the doctor thinks that your baby's head is too big for your pelvis. We think that this is the reason that the baby won't come out.

This diagnosis isn't made because the head is too big for the pelvis necessarily, but because the head is coming into your pelvis cock-eyed (the old *square peg in a round hole* phenomenon). We know that babies stuck in the occiput posterior (OP) position lead to more c-sections because they have a harder time coming through the pelvis that way. We've already talked about how movement and relaxation might help the baby's head come straight into the pelvis. For more on this topic see Chapter Seven.

Large heads usually go hand-in-hand with large babies. We don't really know the size of baby your pelvis can safely deliver until we try. If everything lines up well, a big baby with a big head may fit through just fine. But, if the baby isn't lined up well or is just too big, the baby won't come out. Heroic efforts to make the baby come out could damage your baby's head. Head injuries lead to all sorts of problems, ranging from learning disabilities to cerebral palsy[56].

Doctors and midwives try to make intelligent choices regarding of the safety of attempting vaginal delivery. Most understand the risks of pushing an unlikely situation. If they feel that the head isn't going to come out damage free, they're going to recommend cesarean delivery. And like I've already said, a good cesarean birth is better than a bad vaginal birth.

- ***Shoulder dystocia***

Since we're talking about big babies, let's talk a little about shoulder dystocia. Baby's usually come out sideways, with their shoulders straight up and down along an imaginary line between your pubic bone and your tailbone. If the size of your pelvis and the size of your baby make a tight fit, there's a risk that the top shoulder will get lodged under your pubic bone after the head emerges. This is called shoulder dystocia. It means *stuck*.

Shoulder dystocia tells us that we have a very tight fit on our hands. There are a variety of ideas for avoiding or managing shoulder dystocia, but if it occurs, it's a medical emergency. We work together as a team as quickly as possible, because the risk of injury to the baby goes up the longer the baby is stuck. We only have about 60 seconds to relieve the trapped shoulder before the baby begins to lose oxygen. That may seem like a long time to you, but in the heat of the moment, it feels like an eternity!

Once upon a time I had a mom having her 4th baby. It was her *first* delivery without an epidural. We expected a short labor and easy delivery, and that's exactly what we got—until the head came out. The first thing we do when the head comes out is check to see if the umbilical cord is around the baby's neck. That's the routine. Sometimes we can deliver the baby with the cord around the neck, sometimes we can't. In that case, the cord needs to be clamped and cut while the baby is still inside. Once the cord is cut oxygen flow to baby stops and we need to get the baby out very quickly.

This baby had a very tight cord around her neck. The doctor had to clamp and cut it before delivering the rest of the baby. The next step was to deliver the shoulders. But, when the doctor reached in, she found they were wedged tight. So, now we had a cut cord and stuck shoulders. We implemented all of our maneuvers so quickly our heads were spinning. Even so, the baby didn't come out easily. It took about 45 seconds to get her out. By the time she finally emerged, she was a little stunned. Her first Apgar was 1. But, with a little work, she came around nicely and joined her very happy mommy.

That's shoulder dystocia.

- ***Premature labor***

We've made a lot of guesses as to why some women go into labor before it's time. But the truth is, we really don't know why. We've already talked about why women with twin pregnancies may go into labor early, but all the others are a bit of a mystery. Women can go into labor at any point during their pregnancy.

Obviously, we want to keep the baby in as long as possible. We hope to prevent delivery before the point of viability (about 25 weeks of age). But, every situation is different. If you have premature labor you may be given medication to stop the contractions. Medication for preterm labor can be given by shot, pill or I.V. If you need I.V. medication to stop contractions you'll need to be admitted to the hospital.

Sometimes a day or two of I.V. medication will get things under control and you can be switched to oral medication so you can go home. Sometimes women stay in the hospital on I.V. medication until delivery. Depending upon how far along you are in your pregnancy, you'll also be given a shot of medication to help prepare the baby's lungs for birth. We do this in the event that baby comes despite our best efforts. Two shots of this medication do wonders for helping prepare the baby for breathing.

I've had clients dilated to 4cm as early as 26 weeks of pregnancy. With rest and medication, they were able to get another 10 weeks down the road. This is a fabulous success story, but being in bed that long is really tough. One of our moms coined the phrase, "*Every day's a victory!*" And it is! The longer we can keep baby in the better.

Another thing that's hard for women who've struggled with preterm labor is switching to the delivery pathway when the time comes! If we succeed in keeping the baby in, the realities of true labor take the preterm labor mom off guard. This is because when a woman struggles with preterm labor she's worried about every contraction, fearing that every contraction will make her baby come early.

Once we slow contractions way down, the preterm labor mom will still experience occasional contractions. Five or six an hour are not unusual, but moms still worry about them. We've already talked about how many contractions it takes to get the cervix to dilate progressively. Moms who've spent weeks focusing on every contraction have a hard time believing how many contractions it actually takes to get the cervix to dilate. They've been worried about three contractions an hour, and now we're telling them that they need 20 or 30 an hour to get the cervix to dilate. It can be very confusing.

- ***Breech***

It's rare for providers to deliver vaginally these days if your baby is breech (bottom down). The reason is that the baby's head is the biggest part of the baby. On top of that, the head of a breech baby doesn't have the advantage of *molding* to fit the pelvis through the process of labor. So what we have is a big, round head. The risk that the body will fit through the birth canal but the head won't is frightening. We're in deep water if the body delivers but the head won't.

I'm not going to tell you what they do to get the head out in places of the world where vaginal breech deliveries are done, because it's not pretty. But, because we know what they do, doctors in most developed countries believe that the safest way to deliver a breech baby is by c-section. It may be possible for your doctor to turn your baby a week or two before your due date. Sometimes turning the baby works, sometimes it doesn't.

- *Premature rupture of membranes*
We've talked about this already in Chapter Eight, but it's worth mentioning again. Premature rupture of membranes is when your bag of water breaks *before* labor starts (when you're over 37 weeks). Because the risk for infection goes up with time, your provider will likely recommend inducing labor within 24 hours of your water breaking. Studies demonstrate that inducing labor rather than waiting for labor to start on its own *reduces the risk of uterine infection* and subsequent newborn complications such as cerebral palsy and learning disabilities[26, 28].

- *Fetal intolerance of labor*
We've also talked quite a bit about the baby in labor. This is just a quick review.
There are a lot of reasons why babies don't tolerate labor sometimes. Most of them have to do with *flow* issues like we talked about in Chapter Five. Some flow issues are caused by damage to the placenta from diseases such as preeclampsia or diabetes. Some are caused by overstimulation of the uterus from excessive use of oxytocin. Here's a short list of some other things that may contribute to your baby's inability to tolerate labor:

- Cord around the baby's neck
- Cord wrapped around an arm or leg
- Skinny, short, or knotted cord
- Odd implantation of the cord
- Small, old or injured placenta
- Premature separation of the placenta
- Low levels of amniotic fluid
- Infection
- Premature baby

- Baby with cardiac or neurologic problem
- Prolonged labor or pushing stage

Those of us who care for moms and babies understand that pregnancy is not only wonderful, but that it's also unpredictable. Thankfully, we have excellent obstetric services in most parts of the United States these days, and most complications can be managed quite successfully. If you face an issue with your pregnancy that leads to an experience that you don't want, my heart goes out to you. No woman wants unexpected challenges with her pregnancy, but I'm confident that you'll be well cared for. Our goal is the same as yours; a happy ending to your trying journey.

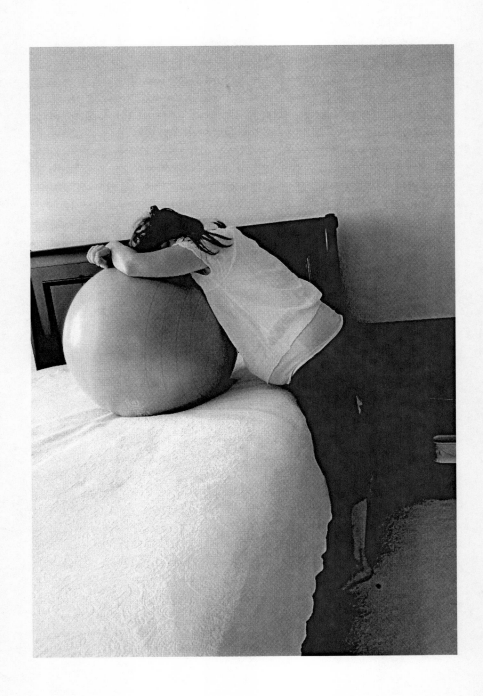

Chapter Twelve
A lively conversation

If you're new to the world of childbirth you might not be aware of the lively conversation taking place out there. But, it won't take you long to learn that there are opinions on every topic! Ever since the beginning of modern obstetrics and the slow shift toward physician run care, people have been debating the best way to care for moms and babies. No one can argue, though, that good things began to happen, even if we disagree over who should get the credit.

In the early 1900's, about 8 women out of every 1000 died of pregnancy related complications in the United States, and 10% of babies didn't live to see their first birthday. Put another way, everyone knew someone who had lost a loved one. Between 1900 and 1997, we've seen dramatic improvement in the numbers. The maternal mortality rate has dropped nearly 99%, and the infant mortality rate more than 90%[27].

The people who've dedicated their lives to this business have strong feelings about the best way to do things, but they don't always agree. Differences of opinion have caused divisions and providers co-exist in various states of harmony; a bit like Republicans and Democrats. Instead of being all bad though, differences can motivate us toward making things better. That's the American way.

Many of you are trying to come to your own conclusions. If you've been exploring the internet you could be feeling a little overwhelmed. The wide range of opinions, from when to cut the cord to whether to have an epidural, can leave you feeling dazed. One of the problems I've noticed, as I've browsed the conversations, is that there seems to be an attempt to package childbirth. Some writers create the impression that the ideal experience is available to all; that all you have to do is take charge and it can be yours. Even though intentions are good, the full picture is often missing.

In this chapter, I'm going to share my thoughts on one of the biggest questions facing women: *Where should I deliver my baby?* Of all the decisions that you'll have to make, this is the most important. Because this decision can be so emotional, it can be difficult to sort out all the issues. What I hope to do is clear away the confusion and offer you some hard-earned wisdom.

Where it all began

Websites and blogs abound with romantic ideas about birth as it used to be, unmolested and untainted by modern medicine. Many of these ideas began sprouting when certain well-meaning women of Hollywood began praising the virtues of out-of-hospital birth and criticizing hospital birth. And as Hollywood goes, so goes the rest of the nation! Hospitals were depicted as insensitive, money-hungry institutions that force their will on women. And, as a result, more and more women have been pursuing out-of-hospital birth, some more successfully than others.

Most of you aren't looking for alternative ideas or words of wisdom. You know that you want to deliver at the hospital because you want what the hospital has to offer, namely an epidural.

But a growing number of you are rethinking your options. I've talked to many women just like you. Intelligent, educated, motivated women. You're considering other options because you *don't* want what the hospital has to offer—whether you know from personal experience or because of the rumors that you've heard.

The primary reason why women consider delivering outside of the hospital is that they've come to believe that the hospital package works against the natural process. They want care takers who believe in normal birth. They want more control and they want people around them who can offer creative ideas and support their dream of a natural labor. Many believe that modern obstetrics has lost track of the ancient art of caring for laboring women as evidenced by the skyrocketing c-section rate. Whether any of these statements about hospitals are true or not, this is how many women feel.

If you're someone who's come to believe that hospital birth is "bad," it might surprise you to learn that I sympathize with many of your concerns. Hospitals have room to grow and I appreciate a thinking population challenging us to take a second look. As I share some thoughts from both sides of the conversation, I'll offer my own opinion on ways that I think hospitals can improve. I'll also share why I think hospital birth is still the best and right option for having a baby.

How are we different from Europe?

Buried deep in the conversation is the secret belief that our system would be much better if it was more like Europe's. Many European women deliver under the care of a midwife in the comfort of their home or in a birthing unit. Women in the U.S. who choose to deliver outside of the hospital believe they're choosing an option parallel to the European model. The problem is that very few parallels exist because our systems are so different.

The European model is midwifery-driven; most obstetricians operate in a consulting role. Women are cared for by midwives during the prenatal period and throughout their labor and delivery. In the U.S. and Canada the majority of women are cared for by physicians throughout their pregnancy and a nurse during their labor. The role of the labor nurse is identical to the role of the European midwife in caring for women during the process of labor, but the actual birth is performed by the physician or midwife.

For many of you the European model as I've just described it makes a great deal of sense and validates your desire for a midwife-managed out-of-hospital birth.

One of the great differences between the American system and the European system is the relationship between physicians and midwives who deliver outside of the hospital.$_{57}$. European midwives delivering outside of the hospital and hospital physicians are partners in care. They have an officially established relationship. This isn't true of the U.S. model. In the vast majority of cases no formal relationship exists between hospital physicians and out-of-hospital midwives. And this lack of relationship can lead to significant problems should an issue during labor arise.

Because the European model is midwifery-driven, there's an established system for transferring a woman to the hospital should transfer become necessary. Many women in the U.S. are led to believe that transfer is easy. You just get in the car or call an ambulance and head to the nearest hospital. The problem is that unless the birth center is a legitimate part of the hospital, the hospital staff knows nothing about you. Birth center midwives are not even required to make a courtesy phone call if things go wrong.

If the midwife follows professional protocol and asks the nearest on-call physician to accept you and he or she refuses, you'll be forced to move onto the next hospital. This is why, if the midwife has experienced rejection before, she may forgo the phone call. She knows you need help and she wants you at the nearest hospital. So instead of a nice professional transfer occurring, you show up on the doorstep of the hospital unannounced and in desperate need of help.

It isn't that obstetricians are hard-hearted or unsympathetic; it's that they've been burned too many times. Here's how it happens:

Most birth centers in the United States are completely independent entities. They have separate policies and separate review mechanisms. This means that the midwife might make decisions during your labor that the local physician considers unacceptable or even negligent. These practice differences are the reason physicians are reluctant to assume care. And yet they're expected to "take over" and fix the situation if things go haywire. The crisis becomes his or hers to remedy. If the baby is in severe distress on transfer and the outcome is bad (i.e. the baby is injured), it's the physician who gets sued. Why is this? Because the physician carries the bigger insurance policy.

Can you understand why there's tension and reluctance on the part of physicians? Many good obstetricians have lost their practice because of one catastrophic lawsuit. Unfortunately, what may have begun as a cooperative relationship between the local hospital and the local birth center has deteriorated, in many instances, to the point of no relationship.

I'm not implying that traumatic transfers are common, but it only takes one or two to sour the system. How many times have we seen something similar happen in our world? One bad situation changes the world for everyone. This is why coffee cups are now labeled "hot" and three-year-olds get frisked at the airport.

I am saying that you should fully understand the nature of the relationship between your midwife and the nearest obstetrician. Transfers of care are not uncommon—even in Europe. According to one source, nearly 40% of first-time moms in Great Britain are transferred from the birthing unit to the hospital$_{58}$. And it's not just because women have decided that they want an epidural, since only 30% of women in Great Britain get epidural anesthesia$_{59}$. Reasons for transfer are more complicated than that.

Another difference between our model and that of Europe's is standardization of midwifery training. Since midwives lie at the heart of the European system, standardization of education and compliance with hospital policies is the norm. In the United States midwives delivering outside of the hospital follow a variety of educational pathways. And since they practice independently there's no accountability in terms of adherence to established guidelines.

Hospital Birth

Undoubtedly, hospital birth was a little scary in the olden days. Women were strapped to gurneys, knocked unconscious with strong medications, isolated from their babies ... shaved, purged and forced to endure it all without their husbands by their side. The good news is that we don't do any of this anymore! We make great effort these days to make hospital birthing units beautiful. We know that women want to deliver in a place that's warm, welcoming, and comfortable.

Even though we've made a lot of progress, we still have room to grow. Many women who want a natural labor would like to have it in a hospital. And they want doctors and nurses who will bravely and creatively support them in their efforts.

Concern over whether or not doctors and nurses will be supportive of natural labor is only one reason why more women are rethinking hospital birth. Many wonder why we use so much oxytocin and perform so many c-sections. They've been told that we routinely break the bag of water and cut episiotomies. And they're told that we impose these things upon women against their will.

The concerns are valid, but they don't tell the whole story. The truth is, that much of what's "imposed" isn't done so against anyone's will. It's done because it is *desired*. In other words, the desire for an epidural begets continuous monitoring and bed rest and oxytocin and catheters ... Epidurals are certainly optional for the vast majority of women, but placing one imposes certain obligations in regards to care.

With the rise in popularity of epidural anesthesia, a whole new approach to care has evolved. High tech labor means that nurses have responsibilities beyond the expected roles of coaching and comforting. Today's labor nurse is also responsible for monitoring, calculating, measuring and documenting. It's an extremely responsible role and one that we take very seriously. Without a doubt it takes effort to keep track of the art while immersed in the demands of the science.

For those inclined to criticism, it might be enlightening to talk with women in other parts of the globe. Millions of women would give their right arm to have such a paradigm imposed upon them. It's even been suggested that this is one reason why c-section rates are so high in some parts; because a surgical birth guarantees an anesthetized birth. It's important therefore that we look at market forces before we paint the whole system black. A generation of women who want a painless birth have driven the industry toward more interventions. (Many of you are nodding!)

We love our modern comforts and the technologies that enrich our lives, like automobiles and cell phones. Some people believe that these inventions subject us to risk too, but most believe that the advantages outweigh the potential disadvantages. Many women want an epidural even if they're told there could be a downside. They apply the same logic to childbirth that they do to other areas of their lives. They believe that the advantages of epidurals outweigh the potential disadvantages.

But, it's true; many of us are pretty attached to the epidural routine and not as enchanted with the natural process as we should be. Doctors and nurses like the advantages of epidurals. They like comfortable patients and the cooperation that that brings. They like the rest and relaxation that patients get. And nurses appreciate having greater opportunity for getting the doctor or midwife to the room for delivery.

It begins with how we introduce nurses to the profession. I once asked a group of new labor nurses freshly returned from a training seminar how nervous they were made to feel on a scale of 1 to 10. The consensus response was "*15.*" This is the culture. We intentionally put the fear of God in their unspoiled hearts so that they'll take their responsibilities seriously. We owe it to our clients. Though it may seem strange to some of you, epidural anesthesia helps relieve some of this anxiety. It gives nurses a greater sense of control and more flexibility.

We need to do better at helping nurses develop their understanding of the mechanisms of labor. We spend a lot of time talking about complications and documentation requirements and not enough time studying the normal process. Nurses need to know more about the relationship between mom's position and baby's position. They need to understand how positioning and movement can help the baby find a good path. They need more teaching on pushing strategies for helping the baby come straight into the pelvis. And they need more teaching in the art of natural labor support, understanding what to say, and what *not* to say.

If you're hoping for a natural labor in the hospital, don't despair! I have no doubt that you can find lovers of natural childbirth in every hospital across the country. It just may take a little probing. Another option you may want to consider is choosing a hospital midwife for your care. Plenty of obstetricians are supportive of natural labor too, but a midwife may have more opportunity to stay with you during your labor. And the issues of *relationship* and *transfer of care* don't exist with hospital midwives.

It's all right to ask questions. I ask them all the time. I think that we do some things too often or out of habit. It's all right for you to ask for the reasons why decisions are made and advocate for a less hands on approach. You aren't going to offend your care takers. Actually we're pretty used to it! We live in a well-informed generation and people ask questions all the time. Here are a few that I ask:

- Why **do** so many women need oxytocin?
- Why do women need so many exams during labor?
- Why do women stay in bed so long before they have an epidural?
- Why don't we intermittently monitor the baby more often (versus continuous monitoring)?
- Why don't we have more training on positioning for fetal rotation?
- How might we be contributing to the c-section rate?
- And is there anything we can do to help reduce the numbers?

Questions are good. They help us grow. You get to be an active participant in your care. But, I also want to encourage you to trust your care takers. People who work in a hospital are highly educated and highly trained. They care for women in labor every day and they're pretty good at it. I suppose there are bad apples in every bunch, but the beauty of hospital care is that if you feel that you drew a bad one, ask for a new one! It's all right. Ask to speak with the charge nurse. She cares about how you feel. It's very important to the hospital that you feel satisfied with your experience. They want you going out into the world telling everyone what a wonderful experience you had.

Is out-of-hospital birth right for you?

Home birth reflects a longing to preserve childbirth as one of the most normal, natural experiences of womanhood. Women have been delivering their babies in their homes for centuries. It's actually the longest standing venue for birth known to man! Many women have wonderful, safe experiences delivering in their homes or in a birth center and they love telling their stories.

About 1% of women delivered outside of the hospital in 2008; two-thirds at home and one-third in a birth center$_{60}$. Thirteen percent of the home births were unintentional (meaning that they intended to deliver in the hospital but the baby had other ideas!) Out-of-hospital midwives have raised the bar high when it comes to just letting the process happen. For women who want a "hands off" birth experience this is very appealing.

If you're someone who's thinking about delivering your baby outside of the hospital, please join me in digging a little deeper into three important topics. No one can tell you what decision to make. I only hope to offer you some thoughts that may help guide you along your way.

Statistics

Midwives who deliver out-of-hospital screen clients to make sure that they meet "low-risk" criteria. This means that if you have any of the complications discussed in the last chapter you won't be considered *low-risk*. You're also not low-risk if you've had any surgery on your uterus in the past, including a c-section.

Everyone in this business knows, though, that a low-risk situation can turn into a high-risk situation in the span of a heartbeat. The numbers bear this out. Studies show that injury rates and death rates for moms and babies are similar between hospital birth and out-of-hospital birth[60]. This statement might make it seem, then, that out-of-hospital birth is just as safe as hospital birth. Since the numbers are the same they must be equally safe, right?

The problem is that women delivering in the hospital and women delivering outside of the hospital are not the same. If only *low-risk* women deliver outside of the hospital and *all* types of women deliver inside the hospital, you wouldn't expect the numbers to be the same. You'd expect the rates for the out-of-hospital group to be significantly lower. But they're not.

In a recent study looking at planned home births in Missouri, researchers found that there was a significantly greater risk of the baby dying during labor in a planned home birth. Babies delivered by non-nurse midwives were also more likely to suffer seizures immediately after birth. Seizures only happen when babies are stressed during labor. Researchers concluded that planned home birth increases the risk of injury to the baby[61].

Maybe the numbers can be explained by the fact that midwifery training (for non-nurse midwives) lacks standardization. Or the fact that out-of-hospital midwives work independently with no one to question them. (Hospital workers are big believers in the "team" approach to care and the accountability that comes with it.) Lack of standardization and lack of accountability sets people up for one of life's most profound truths: we aren't aware of what we don't know.

Maybe less-experienced midwives have skewed the numbers. It takes a lot of practice to develop expertise in assessing a baby's tolerance of labor. It's easy to miss subtle, abnormal changes in the baby's heartbeat if you haven't had much experience.

Consider the following national statistics for 2008:[6]

- There were 4.2 million live births in the United States
- 8% were attended by midwives (93.9% being certified nurse midwives)
- The majority of certified nurse midwives delivered their clients *in* the hospital
- 42,746 women delivered *outside* of the hospital

- Almost 100% of non-nurse midwives delivered out-side of the hospital
- There are approximately 1800 non-nurse midwives in the U.S.
- So, on average, each non-nurse midwife delivered 24 babies that year

This means that some non-nurse midwives delivered 40 babies and some delivered only 8. As with anything, practice leads to expertise. Considering the wide range of possible birth scenarios, even for low-risk women, it would be very difficult for anyone to develop expertise delivering only 8 babies a year.

Transfers

Since getting to the hospital is so important if something goes wrong, let's talk a bit more about the issues related to trans-fer of care. When I talk with women who are thinking about an out-of-hospital delivery I ask them what they'll do if some-thing goes wrong. The standard answer is "*go to the hospital.*" As we keep talking, I realize that they can't quite picture what this might mean.

Twelve-percent of women, on average, transfer to the hospi-tal at some point during their experience—either during labor or after delivery[60]. If you're transferred during labor it will mean that either you're in a great deal of pain and want an epidural, or your baby is in trouble. Either way, the trip to the hospital will be a grueling, potentially risky ordeal.

We've already talked about how lack of relationship between your midwife and the hospital physician may put you into a tough situation should a problem arise. If your midwife attempts to secure the help of a physician and is refused, she'll be compelled to keep making phone calls or send you off unan-nounced. Calling an ambulance forces the hospital to receive you, but it doesn't solve the problems that interfere with good care. This practice (of sending patients to the hospital virtually unannounced) may get you the care you need, but it also aggra-vates the tensions.

Unless you're someone who doesn't care much about personal relationships, being the instigator of hospital tension can be rather awkward. The hospital staff will do their best to care for you efficiently and professionally no matter your situation. But, if you arrive in crisis after a failed attempt to deliver outside the hospital, and your crisis is now their crisis, they won't be happy about it. Especially if decisions were made during your care that they feel were negligent.

Here's the biggest problem. If you need to transfer because your baby is in trouble, you can't guarantee making it to the hospital in time to spare your baby lifelong injury (or worse). Everything takes time, and in an emergency time is our worst enemy. It's hard enough getting someone who's *inside* the hospital system down the hall and to the operating room in time to prevent injury to the baby. It takes even more time if you're coming from *outside* the system.

Landing on the doorstep unannounced also poses some problems. Not every hospital has an obstetrician in-house every moment of the day. If you or your baby are in serious trouble and you need a c-section, you may have to wait until the operating room team can get there. Again, time won't be on your side.

All of this also applies if your need for transfer comes *after* your baby is born. The reason for transferring after delivery is either because you're hemorrhaging or because your baby is struggling to breathe. Both situations could be life-threatening. It might not be possible to get you or your baby to the hospital in time to avoid serious injury or even death.

In order for you to make an informed decision you need to know the facts. I'm not trying to scare you or create an unrealistic view of life. These are honest and serious issues. Of course women have wonderful birth experiences outside of the hospital every day, because birth usually goes very well. It *is* a normal life process. But so is death.

Let me try to explain it another way. Think back to when you were in school. Some kids did well *because of* the teacher, and some kids did well *in spite of* the teacher. (You remember; the ones who got good grades without ever trying). On the other hand, some students failed in spite of the best efforts of the teacher, and some failed (sadly) *because of* the teacher.

Truthfully, birth is the same way. When all goes well, we really don't do much. Most good deliveries happen *in spite of* us (even though we like to say they happen *because of* us!) On the other side of the equation, some deliveries are tough in spite of our best efforts. This is the delivery that demands an experienced provider; someone who can keep their wits about them in the middle of a crisis. Lastly, the one that gets people in trouble is the bad delivery that happens *because of* us.

When women talk about their birth experiences I always wonder which scenario applies. Even though many women praise their providers to the hilt, I secretly know that many of those good deliveries happened *in spite of* the provider.

So where am I going with all of this? I'm trying to give you two more things to chew on. One, take the stories you hear from women delivering outside of the hospital with a grain of salt. Just as in the hospital, many deliveries go well *in spite of the person catching your baby*. And two, if you want a good delivery because of your care takers, there's no substitute for expertise and *all necessary emergency supplies*.

Women leaning away from hospital birth find themselves in a conundrum. Most of you are too young to remember riding bikes without helmets and packing 10 kids into the back of the station wagon. We didn't worry about car seats, seat belts, or running around barefoot. My mother couldn't keep tabs on me with a cell phone. (And even I don't remember the days when a mom would send her 10-year-old out the door with a rifle to go get dinner!)

This generation is fixated on safety. I recently saw a news piece in which a local mom was complaining about a neighborhood pond. She had discovered two children hunting for frogs in the brush. She explained how dangerous it was for children to play so near the pond (even though no children had ever drowned there). Neighborhood mothers had been petitioning the city for years to put fences around the ponds, and her discovery of two children in the bushes was evidence of the need.

It was evidence to me of how worried mothers these days have become.

We believe in protecting our children from the "what-ifs" of life. It's why we put them in car seats. It's right and good to protect our children from the "what-ifs" of journeying down the road. But, no journey has greater implications for your child's *entire* life than his or her journey from the womb. This is why, in my heart-of-hearts, I believe in hospital birth. It's not that hospitals are perfect; it's that they have what it takes to give you and your baby the best chance should any unexpected "what-ifs" occur, namely, an operating room.

If you passionately long for a "hands-off," natural labor I fully believe that you can have it in the hospital.

Stories of my own

Yes, I've been on the receiving end when moms come through the door unannounced. It explains my passion. What I've seen and experienced has changed me forever. It's not that anyone means to hurt someone in their care, but poor judgment and inexperience have lead to some pretty sad situations. It's fair to say that sad situations have happened in the hospital, too, but in the hospital the high level of accountability guards providers from losing sight of what's important.

It was late at night when the phone rang. We were just finishing a c-section for a woman who had a placenta previa and all the rooms were full. The emergency room charge nurse called to say she was sending up a woman in active labor who had just arrived from the nearby birth center.

Her midwife and husband were with her.

Mary was a first-time mom and had been laboring for 36 hours—half of that time at home, and half at the birth center. She couldn't take it anymore and wanted an epidural. The midwife told me that everything had been going well, but Mary seemed to be stuck at 7cm.

She hadn't made any cervical change in six hours.

Mary was tense and shaking. I calmly helped her to bed and turned her to her side. I did my best to calm her down while I listened for her baby with the monitor. The picture that unfolded on the monitor brought grief to my heart. The baby's heart rate swung wildly between 170 and 60 beats per minute in big smooth waves. It was one of the most ominous heart rate patterns that I've ever seen and I had no idea how long it had been like that.

If we were to have any chance of saving Mary's baby we needed to move quickly. Mary was still 7cm, thus our only option was a c-section. Her baby was in severe distress from hours of unproductive labor and more labor would push her over the brink. It was quite likely that, if her baby survived, she would be brain damaged from lack of oxygen.

We mobilized the team very quickly and within 10 minutes Mary's baby girl was born. She had Apgars of 0, 1, and 3 (at one minute, five minutes and ten minutes of birth respectively). Mary's baby lived, but suffered significant neurologic injury. She would probably never walk and never go to school. The future before Mary and her husband was full of pain and uncertainty.

Six months after the delivery, the doctor who did the c-section was sued for damages.

***

The doors swung open and a stretcher came flying through. Someone was in a hurry and I soon discovered why. Jill had recently given birth at home, but, as the midwife explained, they were still waiting for her placenta to come out. It was now three hours (and lots of blood) since Jill's baby was born. Jill was as white as the sheet she was wrapped in and unconscious.

We took Jill to the operating room immediately. A stuck placenta means only one thing: the bleeding won't stop until it comes out. If we couldn't get the bleeding to stop quickly, Jill would soon die of total blood loss. She was half-way there when she rolled through the doors.

Jill's blood pressure was 60/30 and her pulse was 155. We worked very quickly. In short order, with medications and special instruments, the doctor was able to get the placenta out. But that didn't pull Jill out of the woods. She had lost so much blood that she developed a life-threatening condition called DIC and dropped into a coma.

After a week in the intensive care unit, Jill finally opened her eyes and looked into the face of her beautiful new son. A week after, that she was well enough to go home.

I'm not sure that the midwife realized how close she came to losing Jill. The first question she asked, on arrival, was if Jill could have a glass of orange juice.

"She's feeling weak," she said.

The only concern she expressed, as we were settling Jill into the intensive care unit, was when we were going to help Jill breastfeed next.

Maybe unspoken anxiety blinded her to the truth of the situation.

In my personal circle, I know seven women who've delivered (or attempted to deliver) outside of the hospital. I know this isn't many, but they're a representative group—all young, healthy, low-risk women.

Only two had the type of deliveries that they were all dreaming of (the two tall ones!). Two of the others also successfully delivered outside the hospital, but not without troubles. One broke her tailbone leading to months of pain and agony, and one hemorrhaged severely after the placenta was delivered. The other three transferred to the hospital. One got an epidural, and two had babies who required admission to the neonatal intensive care unit. One baby needed special care for over a week.

Childbirth is like a flight across the ocean. In most cases it goes very well. If something goes wrong, though, at 30,000 feet, who do you want at the helm? I can still picture Sully Sullenberger landing his airplane on the Hudson River safely delivering all 155 passengers to another day. If your provider lacks the necessary resources, in either education or equipment, the "*what ifs*" of childbirth can haunt you for a lifetime.

Birth under water

A popular, out-of-hospital experience these days is birth under water. Water birth may be lovely for the mom, but it's not so lovely for the baby. Spend as much time in the tub during your labor as you like, but come out for your delivery. Let me explain the reasons why.

To begin with, let's think about the physiology of birth. When the head comes out, where's the baby's chest? Answer: getting the squeeze of its life in the birth canal! If you've seen the birth of a baby, you might remember seeing water leaking out of the baby's nose and mouth as the head came out. This happens because the chest, being tightly squeezed in the vagina, is being compressed in preparation for breathing. Once the chest is delivered it suddenly expands—drawing, enticing, and compelling the baby toward that first life-sustaining breath.

I've been told by water birth advocates that the hydrostatic pressure of the water keeps the baby from taking that first transitional breath under water. It does? And if so, why is that a good thing? Why would we intentionally keep the baby from doing something that he or she is passionately programmed to do? How is that "*natural*"? Some midwives swirl the baby under water for a spell before letting it surface for air. What's the rationale for this? How is that good care? *And where's the research to support it*? The truth is, this is how babies drown[62,63].

Another person once told me that the baby doesn't start breathing until the umbilical cord is cut. If this is what people believe, I suppose I can understand why they keep the baby swirling underwater for a spell after birth. In reality, babies often try to breathe as soon as their head comes out. If the pressure they receive on their chests in the birth canal doesn't hinder their efforts to breathe, the water in the tub won't either.

People observing breathless babies swirling under water use "*breathlessness*" as evidence that babies don't make an effort to breathe until they emerge. I'd like to suggest another reason. It's highly likely that the baby was so shocked by the delivery that it *couldn't* breathe. This is what happens to baby's who come out stressed. They don't breathe. And, if they don't get help quickly their brains will suffer lack of oxygen. If their brains lack oxygen, they'll run the risk of developing learning disabilities or cerebral palsy or worse. Healthy babies who are born with a good heart rate come crying into the world. It's music to our ears.

Another problem is the delivery itself. The actual moment of birth can be tricky. The baby's cord can be around his or her neck or the shoulders can get trapped. These are common occurrences and both are completely unpredictable. No matter what anyone tells you, performing appropriate delivery maneuvers with your bottom deep in water will be nearly impossible to execute. The time it would take to get you out of the tub and into a position more conducive for safe delivery could well lead to an injured baby.

Your bottom deep in water leads to another issue for the person trying to safely deliver your baby. Your provider must lift your baby to air. Unless the water is only several inches deep, the distance your baby must travel to the surface could cause the umbilical cord to snap[64].

All cords are different lengths. If your baby has a short cord (which you won't know until birth), it may not be long enough to get your baby to the surface. Your provider will then need to lift your bottom out of the water, or pull on the cord. If the cord snaps, both you and your baby will begin to hemorrhage immediately. It will be easier to clamp the cord on the baby's side, but trying to get the severed end on your side can be tricky. Often the cord retracts up into your uterus and is hard to get a hold of.

Picture some other realities with me. Imagine for a moment what the water in the tub is like if the pushing stage is done there. During the pushing phase, bleeding is common. So is urinating and passing stool. Bacteria from your skin will begin to reproduce in such a warm, favorable environment[63]. How many of you want your baby swirling in water like that? How many of *you* want to soak in water like that? It may all be natural, but it isn't very sanitary.

You may say, "I'll get out if I have to toilet myself," but I assure you, it's extremely difficult to move around at this stage of labor. And, most moms aren't even aware of the fact that they have to go to the bathroom. With all the pressure women feel down there, these things just happen.

Lastly, there are no studies that say that your child will be happier, calmer or have a less stressful life if he or she is born in water. Actually there are no studies, as of yet, saying that being born under water benefits your baby in any way[61]. Water birth is strictly an experience that benefits the mother.

Hospitals have been criticized for being a business. Delivering babies is certainly a business, and water birth is a popular sales strategy. It's unlikely that someone is going to tell you about the difficulties they've experienced trying to accomplish a safe birth in the tub if this is what you're shopping for. Many women think that they want to deliver in water because of what they've heard, and there are many people willing to accommodate them. This takes us back to the fact that we've come to the place in our history where we've, unknowingly, placed the *experience* of childbirth above the *goal* of childbirth.

Unassisted childbirth

The latest fad on the market is self-birth. It's a real swing in the pendulum away from the culture of interventions. But it's more than that. Women promoting self-birth are immersed in the belief that delivering their own baby is one of life's most supreme spiritual experiences. They've concocted the romantic notion that being one with themselves, one with the universe, and one with their emerging child bonds them together in some intangible divine union.

It almost goes back to the old Gnostic belief that says that the spiritual realm is the only valid reality; that the physical is only an evil quirk of our imagination. But childbirth, for all its spiritual qualities, is a very physical experience, subject to all the evil quirks of our physical bodies. Women who forget this, forget reality.

Plenty of providers will help you bring your baby out if this is your heart's desire. They'll do the hard part and then let you join in on the easy part. I've worked with several providers (doctors and midwives) who routinely encourage moms to reach down and lift their baby up into their arms. It's a beautiful opportunity. But, laboring on your own and attempting your own delivery without the guidance of a licensed, trained professional lacks the better part of wisdom. (Others might express it a bit differently!) It may even be that if you choose to go it alone and something happens to your baby you could be charged with a crime (i.e. manslaughter, child abuse ...).

The take-home message is *do not consider delivering your baby without the help of a licensed, experienced professional who knows what they're doing.* If you lose your baby, your life will never be the same.

An ideal world

Allow me to dream a little. Wouldn't it be wonderful to live in a world where everyone was happy and we had no problems? To live in a world where *good* news reigned and fear no longer plagued our hearts. This is the dream that binds us heart-to-heart in search of a better world.

I have dreams for the world of childbirth too. I wish that birth was risk-free and that problems never happened. Without problems care providers could live without fear of litigation. Without fear of litigation charting would take on a whole new meaning. Without the need for charting a nurse could spend more time focusing more on the art of care rather than on the details of documentation.

And how different our training would be! Rather than instilling fear into the hearts of our wonderful new nurses, we could spend more time helping them appreciate the wonder of the birth process. We'd be able to help them understand the nuances of labor rather than the nuances of sentence structure.

Each one of us knows that for all our dreams the world we live in is an imperfect place. As much as we want things to always go our way, the world is fraught with hard realities. Childbirth is the worst time to discover this.

It's my hope, that as we've explored the wonders of childbirth together, you've developed a deeper appreciation for the joys as well as the challenges. My greatest dream is that you won't forget the *goal* of childbirth as you plan for the *experience* of childbirth. If you accomplish the *goal* you've had a phenomenal experience!

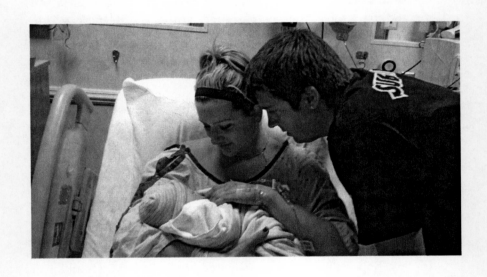

Epilogue

Babette and her beautiful, new son snuggled peacefully together under the warming blanket. Her husband and mom rested quietly in the corner. The week had taken its toll on all of them. Babette started contracting on Monday and was finally admitted to the hospital in labor early Thursday morning. Friday evening at 4pm she delivered a gorgeous 8 pound 10 ounce boy by low transverse c-section. After 4 hours of pushing and a failed attempt to deliver the baby by forceps, the decision to deliver by c-section was made. Babette and her husband were in full agreement.

Friends began filtering quietly through the door, joy and excitement written on their faces. One by one they reached forward to give Babette a kiss on the cheek and coo at her handsome new son. As the last one leaned forward I heard her whisper, "Sweetie, I'm so sorry God didn't answer my prayers. I was so hoping you'd have a normal delivery."

I lifted my eyes from my paperwork and looked over at Babette. The expression in her eyes confirmed my fears. Once we had the room to ourselves again I'd see what I could do to salve the wound that now churned in her heart. Whether she knew it or not, Babette was soon to emerge into a world that puts a grade on childbirth. No one means to do it. Most don't even recognize the new way of thinking. In today's world it seems that the process has become just as important as the prize.

I said a prayer of my own for Babette. She was so tired she didn't have energy to deal with much more stress. As those words would continue to haunt her, I hoped she'd have the wisdom to let them go. I prayed she wouldn't fall into the trap of believing that somehow she was a second-class birther because she delivered by c-section. I also hoped she could be kind to those well-meaning friends who didn't quite see things clearly!

What do we do with disappointment? What do we do when things don't go the way we wanted them to? I'm not talking to those of you who have reason for legitimate sorrow. I've walked this earth long enough to know that some of you have been through painful loss and tragedy. Your journey will take you through deep valleys and dark nights. The support and help you'll need is beyond the scope of this book. But, I certainly can say that help is out there and you need to go after it. Don't let your tragedy be the end of your life. Believe it or not, tragedy in the realm of pregnancy and childbirth unites more women than any other form of earthly calamity. As broken as you are, you're not alone.

But for those of you who went home with a gorgeous, healthy baby you have every reason to hold your head high. Cease grieving that the experience didn't go exactly as you hoped it would. It may be that you wound up at the hospital and gave up on your dream of a home birth. Maybe you broke down and got an epidural after spending weeks practicing natural labor strategies. Or maybe your cervix wouldn't budge past 5cm and you delivered by c-section. Please don't feel guilty, and don't let others make you feel guilty either. Loved ones don't mean to disparage the happiest day of your life; they just need a little education.

Let me offer you a few token pieces of advice to help you through your journey:

1. Realize that you didn't have all the information when you made all your plans. In essence, the decisions that you made *before* labor were not fully informed. The vast majority of women discover that labor is harder than they imagined. Give yourself a break. You are not a failure, and you're not a second-class woman if you changed your mind or ran up against an insurmountable challenge.

2. It's possible that things would have concluded just as they did even if things had been done differently. You may have faced a number of variables that you didn't have any control over. Labor is like that. Please don't beat yourself up over the "what-ifs." Life's too short. And the good news is that second labors are usually easier! Try again for that natural labor the next time around.

3. Childbirth is only one day in your life. Remember, you weren't planning for a day; you were planning for a relationship.

Moving on

If you're someone who feels bad about your experience, you'll need to find a way to overcome your disappointment and move on. Don't let anger or bitterness take root in your heart. Without realizing it, your sorrow can seep into all your special relationships, even your relationship with your child. You want to be the kind of person who can teach your child how to overcome adversity and deal with disappointment. This is how you'll help him or her become strong and successful. So, look at your sweet baby and cultivate thankfulness.

Parenting is a wonderful adventure. Look to the joy of your future, and consider yourself blessed if you have a beautiful new person to share it with.

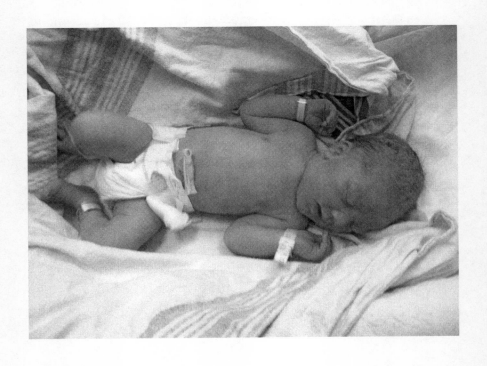

Endnotes

1. Simpson, K.R. (2008). Labor and Birth. In K.R. Simpson & P.A. Creehan, (Eds.), *Perinatal nursing*, 3rd ed., New York: Lippincott, Williams & Wilkins.

2. Centers for Disease Control and Prevention. (2010). *Group B Strep (GBS)*. Fast Facts. Retrieved February 4, 2012, from www.cdc.gov/groupbstrep/about/fast-facts.html

3. *As a man thinketh.* (n.d.). Retrieved December 5, 2011, from Wikipedia http://en.wikipedia.org

4. World Health Organization. (2011). *Maternal mortality ratio.* Global Health Observatory Data Repository. Retrieved May 7, 2012, from http://apps.who.int/ghodata/?vid=93000

5. Scientific Advisory Committee on Nutrition. (2011). *The influence of maternal, fetal, and child nutrition on the development of chronic disease later in life.* Retrieved from www.sacn.gov.uk/pdfs/sacn_early_nutrition_final_report_20_6_11.pdf

6. Sutton, J., Scott, P. (1996). *Understanding and teaching optimal foetal positioning*, 2nd ed., Birth Concepts: Tauranga, New Zeland.

7. *Beefalo.* (n.d.). Retrieved December 9, 2011, from Wikipedia www.en.wikipedia.org

8. Simkin, P., Bolding, A. (2004). Update on nonpharmacologic approaches to relieve labor pain and prevent suffering. *Journal of midwifery & women's health, 49*(6), 489–504.

9. Zwelling, E. (2010). Overcoming the challenges: maternal movement and positioning to facilitate labor progress. *MCN. The American Journal of Maternal Child Nursing, 35*(2), 72–78.

10. Gilbert, J.G. (2012). *Pharmacologic management of pain during labor and delivery.* Retrieved May 19, 2012, from www.uptodate.com

11. Moffat, F.W., Feinstein, N. (2003). Techniques for fetal heart assessment. In Feinstein, N., Torgersen, K.L., Atterbury, J. (Eds.), *AWHONN: Fetal heart monitoring principles and practices.*, 3rd ed., Dubuque: Kendall/Hunt Publishing Company.

12. Goetzl, L.M. (2002). *Obstetric analgesia and anesthesia: Clinical management guidelines for Obstetrician-Gynecologists*, ACOG Practice Bulletin, Number 36. Retrieved from http://www.ncbi.nlm.nih.gov/pubmed/12100826

13. Courtney, K. (2007). Maternal anesthesia: what are the effects on neonates? *Nursing for women's health, 11*(5), 499–502.
14. Lusskin, S.I., Misri, S. (2011). *Postpartum blues and depression.* Retrieved July 15, 2012, from www.uptodate.com
15. Khadilkar A, Odebiyi DO, Brosseau L, Wells GA. *Transcutaneous electrical nerve stimulation (TENS) versus placebo for chronic low-back pain.* Cochrane Database of Systematic Reviews 2008, Issue 4. Art. No.: CD003008. DOI: 10.1002/14651858.CD003008.pub3.
16. Simkin, P., Klein, M.C. (2012). *Nonpharmacological approaches to management of labor pain.* Retrieved May 20, 2012, from www. uptodate.com
17. Loubert, C., Hinova, A., Fernando, R. (2011). Update on modern neuraxial analgesia in labour: A review of the literature of the last 5 years. *Anaesthesia, 66,* 191–212.
18. Satpathy, H.K. (2011). Labor and deliver, analgesia, regional and local. Retrieved June 13, 2012, from www.emedicine.medscape.com
19. Gilbert, J.G. (2012). *Neuraxial analgesia and anesthesia for labor and delivery: Options.* Retrieved June 5, 2012, from www.uptodate.com
20. Cambic, C.R., Wong, C.A. (2010). Labour analgesia and obstetric outcomes. *British Journal of Anaesthesia, 105*(1), 50–60.
21. Briggs, G.G., Wan, S.R. (2006). Drug therapy during labor and delivery, part 2. *American Society of Health-system Pharmacists, 63,* 1131–1139.
22. Capogna, G., Camorcia, M. (2004). Epidural analgesia for childbirth: Effects of newer techniques on neonatal outcomes. *Pediatric drugs, 6*(6), 375–386.
23. Anim-Somuah, M., Smyth, R.M.D, Jones L. *Epidural versus non-epidural or no analgesia in labour.* Cochrane Database of Systematic Reviews 2011, Issue 12. Art. No.: CD000331. DOI: 10.1002/14651858.CD000331.pub3.
24. Declercq, E., Menacker, F., MacDorman, M., (2006). Maternal risk profiles and the primary cesarean rate in the United States, 1991–2002. *American Journal of Public Health, 96*(5), 867–872.
25. National Center for Health Statistics: National Vital Statistics Report. (2007). *Fetal and perinatal mortality, 56*(3).
26. Jazayeri, A. (2011). *Premature rupture of membranes.* Retrieved August 1, 2012, from www.emedicine.medscape.com

27. Centers for Disease Control. (1999). Achievements in Public Health, 1900–1999: Healthier mothers and babies. MMWR Weekly, 48(38), 849–858.

28. Sherman, M.P. (2011). *Chorioamnionitis.* Retrieved July 31, 2012, from www.emedicine.medscape.com

29. Lowdermilk, D.L., Perry, S.E. (2007). *Maternity & Women's Health Care.* 9th ed., Mosby Elsevier: St. Louis.

30. Wing, D.A. (2012). *Principles of labor induction.* Retrieved May 3, 2012, from www.uptodate.com

31. The American Congress of Obstetricians and Gynecologists. (2011, December). *Optimizing protocols in obstetrics: Oxytocin for induction.* ACOG Practice Bulletin, *114*(2).

32. Weiss, R.E. (n.d.). *5 ways Pitocin is different from oxytocin.* Retrieved July 18, 2012, from www.pregnancy.about.com

33. *Oxytocin.* (n.d.). Retrieved July 16, 2012, from Wikipedia www. en.wikipedia.org/wiki/Oxytocin

34. Balasch, J., Gratacos, E. (2012). *Delayed childbearing: Effects on fertility and the outcome of pregnancy.* Current Opinion in Obstetrics & Gynecology, *24*(3), 187–193.

35. Ogden, C.L., Carroll, M.D., Kit, B.K., Flegal, K.M. (2012). Prevalence of obesity in the United States, 2009–2010. *NCHS Data Brief,* 82, Centers for Disease Control.

36. Bayrampour, H., Heaman, M. (2010). Advanced maternal age and the risk of cesarean birth: A systematic review. *Birth: Issues in Perinatal Care.* 37(3), 219–26.

37. World Health Organization, UNICEF, UNFPA, and The World Bank. (2012). *Trends in maternal mortality: 1990 to 2010.* Retrieved August 13, 2012, from World Health Organization, http://www. unfpa.org/public/home/publications/pid/10728

38. Gibbons, L., Belizan, J.M., Lauer, J.A., Betran, A.P., Merialdi, M., Althabe, F. (2010). The global numbers and cost of additionally needed and unnecessary caesarean sections performed per year: Overuse as a universal barrier to coverage. World Health Report, Background paper 30. World Health Organization.

39. Frequently asked questions about midwives and midwifery. (n.d.). Retrieved March 17, 2012 from Citizens for midwifery. www. cfmidwifery.org

40. *Current status.* (n.d.). Retrieved March 17, 2012, from North American Registry for Midwives. www.narm.org

41. *Our credentials.* (n.d.). Retrieved March 17, 2012, from American College of Nurse-Midwives. www.midwife.org

42. *Midwives.* (n.d.). Retrieved March 17, 2012, from www.kidshealth.org

43. *Doula.* (n.d.). Retrieved March 21, 2012, from Wikipedia. http://en.wikipedia.org/wiki/Doula

44. Stuebe, A., Barbieri, R.L. (2011). *Continuous intrapartum support.* Retrieved January 3, 2012, from www.uptodate.com

45. Barron, M.L. (2008). Antenatal Care. In K.R. Simpson & P.A. Creehan, (Eds.), *Perinatal nursing,* 3rd ed., New York: Lippincott, Williams & Wilkins.

46. August, P., Sibai, B. (2012). *Preeclampsia: Clinical features and diagnosis.* Retrieved June 5, 2012, from www.uptodate.com

47. Magloire, L., Funai, E.F. (2011). *Gestational hypertension.* Retrieved May 22, 2012, from www.uptodate.com

48. Jovanovic, L. (2011). *Patient information: Gestational diabetes mellitus (Beyond the Basics).* Retrieved June 11, 2012, from www.uptodate.com

49. Caughey, A.B. (2012). *Obstetrical management of pregnancies complicated by gestational diabetes mellitus.* Retrieved June 28, 2012, from www.uptodate.com

50. Martin J. A., Hamilton B. E., Osterman M.J.K. (2012). *Three decades of twin birth in the United States, 1980–2009.* National Center for Health Statistics Data Brief No. 80.

51. Smith, G.C.S., Fleming, K.M., White, I.R. (2007). Birth order of twins and risk of perinatal death related to delivery in England, Northern Ireland, and Wales, 1994–2003: Retrospective cohort study. *BMJ;*334:576.

52. Yang, X., Kellems, R.E. (2009). Is preeclampsia an autoimmune disease? *Clinical immunology, 133*(1), 1–12.

53. Magann, E.R., Doherty, D.A., Briery, C.M., Niederhauser, A., Morrison, J.C. (2006). Timing of placental delivery to prevent post-partum haemorrhage: Lessons learned from an abandoned randomised clinical trial. *Australian and New Zealand Journal of Obstetrics and Gynaecology, 46:* 549–551.

54. Doumouchtsis, S.K., Arulkumaran, S. (2010). The morbidly adherent placenta: An overview of management options. *Acta Obstetricia et Gynecologica. 89:* 1126–1133.

55. Smith, J.R. (2012). Management of the third stage of labor. Retrieved August 1, 2012, from www.emedicine.medscape.com

56. Kopelman, A.E. (2009). Birth injury. *The Merck Manual Home Health Handbook.* Retrieved June 13, 2012, from www.merckmanuals.com

57. British Council. (2005). *Nursing and midwifery.* Retrieved March 6, 2012, from www.britishcouncil.org/learning-infosheets-nursing.pdf.

58. *All about birth centres.* (2010). Retrieved June 22, 2012, from www.babycentre.co.uk/pregnancy

59. *Epidural.* (2012). Retrieved June 22, 2012, from www.babycentre.co.uk

60. Declerq, E., Stotland, N.E. (2011). *Planned home birth.* Retrieved February 1, 2012, from www.uptodate.com

61. Chang, J.J., Macones, G.A. (2011). Birth outcomes of planned homes births in Missouri: A population-based study. *American Journal of Perinatology, 28*(7), 529–536.

62. Batton, D.G., Blackmon, L.R., Adamkin, D.H., Bell, E.F., Denson, S.E., Engle, W.A., … Couto, J. (2005). Underwater births. *Pediatrics, 115*(5), 1413–1414.

63. Byard, R.W., Zuccollo, J.M. (2010). Forensic issues in cases of water birth fatalities. *The American Journal of Forensic Medicine and Pathology, 31*(3), 258–260.

64. *Water birth.* (2007). Retrieved September 10, 2012, from American Pregnancy Association www.americanpregnancy.org

Appendix
Self-evaluation

1. I'm an overachiever.

No, this doesn't describe me.	1 2 3 4 5	Yes, this describes me to a tee!

2. I'm prone to feeling guilty.

No, this doesn't describe me.	1 2 3 4 5	Yes, this describes me to a tee!

3. I'm very competitive.

No, this doesn't describe me.	1 2 3 4 5	Yes, this describes me to a tee!

4. I frequently compare myself to other women.

No, this doesn't describe me.	1 2 3 4 5	Yes, this describes me to a tee!

5. I want the kind of birth experience that my friend "_____" had.

No, this doesn't describe me.	1 2 3 4 5	Yes, this describes me to a tee!

Assuming a healthy baby and a healthy mommy, your score might reveal how you'll respond emotionally if your birth experience doesn't go exactly like you hope.

Score 20-25:	You might feel depressed if your birth experience doesn't go exactly like you hope.
Score 15-19:	You might feel disappointed if your birth experience doesn't go exacly like you hope.
Score 10-14:	You'll be ok if things go exactly like you hope.
Score 5-9:	You'll be happy with any experience as long as you have a healthy baby in your arms.

Packing for the hospital

- Insurance information
- Comfortable clothes for everyone
- Slippers
- Outfit to take the baby home in
- Baby blanket
- Car seat
- Phone numbers
- Camera
- Snacks: real food for dad, favorite popsicles for mom
- Favorite pillow

If you forget something, someone can go back and get it for you later. Don't spend time running around the house to get something if you really need to be on your way. They have everything you need at the hospital.

Writing a birth plan

You now know my perspective on birth plans. The vast majority of women don't write one, and you don't need one to have a good experience. But if you feel the need to write one, keep it simple. Here are some ideas that might be helpful:

- Tell us a little about yourself
- What kind of experience are you hoping for?
- If you're hoping for a natural labor, how committed are you to this goal?
- Do you have any particular things that you'd like to do or try during your labor? Your pushing stage?
- What kind of atmosphere would you like us to help create?
- Who can we expect in the room with you?
- What strategies have you been preparing?
- How would you like us to participate?
- How many ideas or strategies would you like us to suggest?
- How much would you like us to encourage you through the hard parts?
- What should we do if you say that you want to change your mind?
- What will the "code" be that you really do want to change your mind?
- Are you someone who will need encouragement if you do change your mind?

A special thank you to everyone who helped to create the photographic artwork: Ryan, Missy and Caiden McCarthy, Olapeju Ogunyemi, Kristi Robinson, and last, but not least, Rita the Red-Head.

If you have a question, or would like to share your thoughts with me, I can be reached at laboringwell@gmail.com.

CPSIA information can be obtained at www.ICGtesting.com
Printed in the USA
BVOW070639070213

312607BV00002B/69/P